Understanding Regulation Disorders of Sensory Processing in Children

of related interest

Understanding Sensory Dysfunction
Learning, Development and Sensory Dysfunction in Autism Spectrum Disorders,
ADHD, Learning Disabilities and Bipolar Disorder
Polly Godwin Emmons and Liz McKendry Anderson
ISBN: 978 184310 806 1

Living Sensationally
Understanding Your Senses
Winnie Dunn
ISBN 978 184310 871 9

Sensory Smarts
A Book for Kids with ADHD or Autism Spectrum Disorders Struggling with
Sensory Integration Problems
Kathleen A. Chara and Paul J. Chara, Jr.
With Christian P. Chara
Illustrated by J.M. Berns
ISBN 978 184310 783 5

Music Therapy, Sensory Integration and the Autistic Child
Dorita S. Berger
Foreword by Donna Williams
ISBN 978 184310 700 2

Sensory Perceptual Issues in Autism and Asperger's Syndrome
Different Sensory Experiences, Different Perceptual Worlds
Olga Bogdashina
Forewords by Wendy Lawson and Theo Peeters
ISBN 978 184310 166 6

Kids in the Syndrome Mix of ADHD, LD, Asperger's, Tourette's, Bipolar, and More!
The one stop guide for parents, teachers and other professionals.
Martin L. Kutscher MD
With a contribuition from Tony Attwood
With a contribution from Robert R Wolff MD
Hardback ISBN 978 184310 810 8

Practical Sensory Programmes for Students with Autism Spectrum Disorder
and Other Special Needs
Sue Larkey
ISBN 978 184310 479 7

Integrated Yoga
Yoga with a Sensory Integrative Approach
Nicole Cuomo
ISBN 978 184310 862 7

Understanding Regulation Disorders of Sensory Processing in Children

Management Strategies for Parents and Professionals

Pratibha Reebye and Aileen Stalker

Jessica Kingsley Publishers
London and Philadelphia

First published in 2008
by Jessica Kingsley Publishers
116 Pentonville Road
London N1 9JB, UK
and
400 Market Street, Suite 400
Philadelphia, PA 19106, USA

www.jkp.com

Copyright © Pratibha Reebye and Aileen Stalker 2008

Photographs on pp.31, 33, 43(a), 52(a), 88, 92 © Tim and Anna Hippmann 2008
Photographs on pp.43(b), 59, 62, 67, 74, 81(b), 86, 97, 99, 106, 114 © Aileen Stalker 2008
Photographs on pp.52(b), 64, 71(b), 133, 144 © Pratibha Reebye 2008
Photographs on pp.71(a), 81(a) © Jeanette and Ulrich Paschen 2008

Library of Congress Cataloging in Publication Data
A CIP catalog record for this book is available from the Library of Congress

British Library Cataloguing in Publication Data
A CIP catalogue record for this book is available from the British Library

ISBN 978 1 84310 521 3

Printed and Bound in the United States by
Thomson-Shore, Inc.

This book is dedicated to the children and parents of children with Regulation Disorders of Sensory Processing from whom we learned so much, and to our own families, Patrick and Andrew Nolan (Aileen), Rajiv, Uday and Smita and husband Nittin (Pratibha).

CONTENTS

ACKNOWLEDGMENTS

One of the newest diagnoses given to children who are assessed and treated within infant mental health and developmental clinics is that of Regulation Disorders of Sensory Processing (RDSP). Parents, caregivers, educators and health practitioners often feel uninformed, unsupported and alone in their quest to provide the best learning and living environments for the children identified as having this disorder. Unfortunately, when these children are not appropriately identified and do not receive timely supports and intervention, their development may be at risk. It was when working with groups of parents of children with RDSP that the need for this type of book became apparent. The parents received support and information within the group, but expressed the need for written information to share with family members, educators, medical professionals and community staff. The willingness of these parents to share their ideas, feelings and strategies provided real-life input into the suggestions within this book. Their dedication and patience with their children provided inspiration and hope to other parents and to us. And, because we truly believe that all children deserve a community of people who love and encourage them, we hope that when you read this book, whether you are a parent, relative, teacher, health professional or community worker, you will think of the children that you know who have RDSP and benefit from the combined expertise of parents and professionals that helped to provide the ideas within this book. We would also like to thank our families and colleagues who encouraged our efforts in developing this book, and who gave valuable feedback and unfailing support. The beautiful babies, toddlers and children in the pictures are children of our friends and who attend Shannon Daycare, who smiled and cried and were regular kids while being photographed.

Part One

UNDERSTANDING REGULATION DISORDERS

Chapter 1

INTRODUCTION

What are Regulation Disorders of Sensory Processing?

Human infants are able to maintain an internal equilibrium by modulating sensory stimulation from the environment. Their regulation capacities include the ability to modulate the intensity of arousal experienced while remaining engaged in an interaction or being able to disengage easily from an activity.

Regulation capacities increase with age and by age six most children have learned to adjust their behaviors and sensory needs. However, infants and toddlers with Regulation Disorders (RDSP) may continue to have mild to intense difficulties in some areas of their sensory, motor and behavioral regulation throughout their childhood.

It was recognition of the persistent characteristics of these difficulties that established Regulation Disorders of Sensory Processing (RDSP) as a diagnostic category within early childhood disorders. The presence of sensory reactivity, motor and behavioral patterns across settings and within multiple relationships characterize this disorder (Diagnostic Catergory [DC]: 0–3R, ZERO TO THREE 2005).

Long before a clinical diagnosis is made, astute parents of a child with RDSP have observed that their child does not react like other children of the same age, or how their siblings responded at a similar age. Questions the parents may ask before they received a diagnosis are: "Is there something really wrong? Is it a phase? Is it just my child's temperament? My child is really bright; how can there be this other aspect to his behavior and reactions? Do I have to place him in a specialized school environment? How can I help him to have joy in his life?"

Parents' own instincts that there is something unusual with their child's responses are often negated by those around them. Friends, relatives, and passing strangers frequently offer their advice and observations about the cause of the child's behaviors, saying, "Have another one and that will sort him out", "It's your first child…", "You are spoiling your child", "You are doing it wrong", "You are over-focusing because he is the first boy…"

Medical professionals may respond by suggesting it is a stage the child is going through or that the child will "grow out of it."

However, parental descriptions of their children indicate a spectrum of symptoms that exceed those of typically responding children.

During infancy, parents describe their children as active, fussy, rigid, and having excessive crying, sleep problems, eating problems and touch sensitivity, as well as experiencing "colic-like" behaviors for their whole infancy. These babies are ones that need complete darkness to sleep, need to be driven around in a car for the vibration or "white noise" effect to help them calm, and are hypersensitive to sound and images. They may also have difficulty regulating their eating and elimination patterns, and difficulty self-calming generally.

During toddler and preschool years, parents relate that their children demonstrate a lack of awareness of personal space, safety and judging distances, experience tactile and noise sensitivity, fine motor problems, food allergies, excessive movement in sleep, and night terrors. The children sometimes are advanced in cognitive areas but often have poor social skills, seek out and play better with younger or older children and desperately want control of their environment. Although they may be engaging and charming, they can rapidly switch to violent outbursts or reactions manifested as aggression or negativity. Their conversational ability may be high but they may have slow speed in completion of goal-directed activities.

As the children become older preschoolers, the parents report that the children have difficulty tolerating the feeling of certain clothes, have difficulty with temperature control, and may perspire a lot. They want to eat only certain foods, are fearful of the flushing of the toilet, or hate to have their teeth or hair brushed or cut. These children may also become perseverative and get stuck in a play routine, repeating the same play over and over, or only play with certain toys. They may fear the unknown, such as when they see a Santa Claus or a clown, as the distortion of the human image is confusing for them. They may crave the feeling of gravity – and enjoy swinging and rides at amusement parks for long periods of time.

During primary school years, the parents describe that their children have difficulty with transitions, are reactive to noises and touch, and demonstrate more fine and gross motor problems compared to their peers. They may make impulsive responses, which are frequently interpreted as aggressive behavior, and exhibit poor social skills. Because of impulsivity and aggression, it is difficult to include them in shopping or many outside events. Their difficulty with perspective taking and their own bossy and aggressive behaviors result in few sustained friendships. Although they can attend to play for short periods of time, their play then shifts, and may be interrupted by their constant craving for personal attention. The children can not stand to lose face or be wrong, but they can find something wrong in everything. They may have obsessive behaviors where they over-focus or are preoccupied with a certain method or behavior, although they often are verbally adept.

Although parents can describe many troubling aspects of their children, these children are difficult to describe precisely or define because they change from day to day and are complex and individual in their sensory and behavioral responses.

However, to assist professionals and those who work or play with the child, it is often helpful to have a specific diagnosis that matches a clinical description.

A clinical description of Regulation Disorders

In both the International Classification of Diseases (ICD-9-CM) and the Diagnostic and Statistical Manual Text Revised (DSM-IV-TR), there is no description or provision for the diagnosis of Regulation Disorders/Regulation Disorders of Sensory Processing.

This diagnosis is a category in the DC: 0–3R, *Diagnostic Classification of Mental Health and Developmental Disorders of Infancy and Early Childhood*, which is a diagnostic manual produced by the ZERO TO THREE organization. Recently revised (2005), the disorder is now called Regulation Disorders of Sensory Processing, to emphasize that difficulty in sensory processing is a pivotal symptom observed in these disorders.

When establishing the diagnosis within infants, clinicians looked at the babies that used to be called "fussy" or "colicky" babies in infancy and early childhood.

They recognized that the concept of regulation was important and that development of regulation of mood, impulse, and an internal state of regulation was an essential developmental process. When Dr. Georgia DeGangi, Dr. Serena Weider, Dr. Winnie Dunn and Dr. Stanley Greenspan began focusing their work in the area of children under the age of four, they provided insights into the development and interactions of attachment, emotional regulation, and internal regulation. The diagnosis of RDSP has been supported within their research and the research of other clinicians during the last ten years.

RDSP is not designated as a diagnostic category by exclusion (if it is not that, then it is this). It represents a definite entity that requires a distinct behavioral pattern for diagnosis. The diagnosis is not related to a child's intelligence but rather to a pattern of responses and behaviors observed over time. Sensory, motor (gross and fine motor), physiological (sleep, eating and elimination), behavioral processing and organizational (attention and affect, and overall behavior) responses are all considered. (Sleeping and eating difficulties can be considered symptoms of RDSP or as separate problems.) The disorders affect daily adaptation, interactions and relationships (DC: 0–3R 2005).

Regulation Disorders – what causes them?

RDSPs are most evident in infancy and early childhood. The causes are unclear. Each child has his individual sensory, motor, physiological and behavioral processing and organizational pattern and needs. The child with RDSP has more accentuated patterns in one or many of these areas.

Symptoms of infants with RDSP are not static and evolve over time. Early detection may therefore prevent more serious, long-term perceptual, language, sensory integrative and behavioral difficulties. Parents and others involved with the infants or children need to know that RDSPs are multifactorial in origin. The theories range from having an overlap with difficult temperament (DeGangi *et al.* 1993) to speculations about atypical central nervous system functioning.

Parents are often surprised that all the children in their family show some type of regulation difficulties, either sleep, feeding or sensory issues. That observation often gives rise to fears that RDSP may be a genetic disorder. At the time of writing, there are no literature references to support this notion.

The behavioral responses of infants, toddlers and children with RDSP are easily misinterpreted and causes misattributed. The toddler or child with RDSP is not hyperactive, aggressive or oppositional as judged on an overall behavioral response but may demonstrate these behaviors because of difficulty in emotional regulation related to specific sensory responses. They are often on an emotional roller-coaster rather than having persistent negative emotional responses.

Research in the causes and stability of Regulation Disorders

Fortunately, new findings on self-regulation capacities of infants and young children are emerging. Some clues that point toward physiological and central nervous system adaptability are important to discuss. We would like to remind readers that not all the work mentioned here is specific to RDSP. It does, however, help to explain some of the peculiarities and sensitivities exhibited by children with RDSP.

Porges *et al.* (1996) discuss variations in psychophysiology that allow us to understand differential responses that we see clinically among children with RDSP. One example is an inefficient physiological response such as higher cry thresholds and differences in heart-rate variability. Possible sympathetic dominance lowering the infant's threshold for arousal is also implicated (Lester and Boukydis 1990).

In a four-year follow-up of infants with RDSP, higher baseline cardiac vagal tone was associated with poorer developmental, sensory motor and/or emotional and behavioral difficulties, suggesting some relationship between the vagal tone and persistence of RDSP over time (DeGangi *et al.* 1993).

Parents often ask if their child will always have this disorder and how their child will look and act as they get older. At present, there are no research studies that describe the long-term stability of RDSP over time. However, clinical experience indicates that, from ages two to five, RDSP continues to be an appropriate diagnosis. Many of the early symptoms and behavioral responses continue to be demonstrated by the children until about age eight, when they decrease and social skills increase. However, some children at this age have responses that look like Attention Deficit Hyperactivity Disorder (ADHD) behaviors and need help with emotional, attention and impulse control, as well as assistance with social skills. Other children appear similar to children with Asperger's Syndrome but are more able to have intense social behaviors than children with that diagnosis. Children with an under-reactive type of RDSP are often misdiagnosed with the diagnosis of Autism Spectrum Disorder (ASD).

One important clinical question is whether RDSP are a harbinger to later difficulties in a child's life. If so, what could be done to prevent the progression of symptoms?

In a prospective descriptive investigation, DeGangi *et al.* (1993) found that infants with baseline higher scores on cardiac vagal tone persisted with behavioral difficulties and poorer developmental outcome. Then DeGangi and her colleagues considered how the infants with RDSP fared when treatment was offered.

Thirty-nine infants were diagnosed with RDSP through interdisciplinary assessment. These infants were followed and reassessed at three years of age. Of the 39 subjects, 26 chose treatment, and the remaining 13 constituted the untreated group of infants with RDSP. Eleven infants without the diagnosis of RDSP constituted the control group. The finding that infants with RDSP showed more problems than normal control infants regarding sensory integration, regulation, attention, motor, sleep and behavioral difficulties was not surprising. However, the findings that the self-selected treated infant group given 12 weeks of intensive child-centered intervention (sensory integration therapy, parent guidance and parent–child play) did well on emotional and behavioral indicators, in spite of having more sensory and constitutional problems than untreated infants with RDSP, has clinical significance. The finding that treated infants showed more feeding problems and parental depression between 7 and 30 months, compared to the untreated group, could not be explained satisfactorily. At three years, untreated children with RDSP showed more emotional and behavioral problems, and treated children with RDSP had more motor and sensory integrative problems (DeGangi *et al.* 1996).

There are, however, problems with researchers using varying diagnostic criteria in the stability research. Becker *et al.* (2004) found that family adversity seemed more important than multiple regulation difficulties for predicting later hyperkinetic symptoms. These researchers, however, did not use the criteria for RDSP as specified by the DC: 0–3 diagnostic system.

DeGangi *et al.* (2000) carried out another prospective study with two age-matched groups of children aged 7 to 30 months, with RDSP, based on severity of RDSP symptoms. They included ten infants with mild RDSP symptoms, 22 infants with moderate/severe RDSP symptoms, 38 age-matched control infants, and a fourth group of 19 infants diagnosed with Pervasive Developmental Disorder (PDD). At 36 months, 60 percent of the children with mild RDSP identified at 7 and 30 months of age did not meet any criteria for RDSP. (Diagnosis of what was originally called Regulation Disorder was not made using DC: 0–3 criteria since the system was not available at the time of the initial study.) However, 95 percent of infants with moderate RDSP could be identified in two clusters that demonstrated deficits – a motor–language–cognitive development cluster and a parent–child relational cluster. A most interesting observation is that infants initially diagnosed with PDD were given a DSM-IV diagnosis at age 36 months of PDD and cognitive delay. This study also found that children with PDD shared attributes of children with RDSP.

In our follow-up at the British Columbia's Children's Hospital (BCCH) Infant Psychiatry Clinic, there were two points of note. We found that the outcome of RDSP symptoms depended on when we assessed the progression. The majority of children were preschoolers at the time of first diagnosis. At six-months follow-up, a majority of the children no longer demonstrated any symptoms (quit symptoms), but at one-year follow-up there were more problems resembling ASD than ADHD and after two years of follow-up, the majority were either diagnosed as having ADHD or were treated for symptoms of ADHD. Some of the children, at the end of a three-year follow-up, were split into either having a confirmed diagnosis of ADHD or ASD. These clinical observations were for cases seen from 1999 to 2003. They have prompted us to look at our data in a methodical fashion and the analysis of our sample is ongoing. We are moving closer to an answer to the hypothesis regarding whether or not RDSP in which sensory integration difficulties are more prominent seem to be a harbinger to the diagnoses of ADHD or ASD. The exact significance of this phenomenon can only be reported when the analysis of the data is completed.

Prevalence and gender differences in children with Regulation Disorders

There are a greater number of boys than girls with this disorder. In a series of parent groups for parents of children with RDSP, held at BCCH (a tertiary regional paediatric hospital), with the average of six parents per group, only two families with girls were referred.

A chart review completed at BCCH for a period of five years revealed seven girls and 33 boys – a ratio of 4.7 boys to one girl. The children all had reported regulation difficulties, diagnosable by the DC: 0–3 (1994) definition in use at the time.

Similar findings are also reported by Israeli researchers. Tirosh *et al.* (2003) indicated different prevalence depending on the age of the children. Among a younger group (age 6 to 17 months), the statistically significant prevalence among boys was 23.5 percent and girls 13.1 percent. Among the older age group (18 to 36 months) there was a trend with 21.1 percent prevalence among boys and 14.8 percent among the girls.

There is little research on gender differences in behaviors and responses in children with RDSP. Parent observations indicate that girls do not act out with aggressive behaviors as much as boys but often demonstrate high impulsivity that may result in danger to themselves. Girls appear to have more difficulty shifting mental set (thinking about new information or mentally moving back and forth between information content) and with transitions. They may not be aggressive to others but often are towards themselves. Boys may have more behavioral and attention problems. They may be more inept in motor areas and more physically aggressive. Boys may have more expressive language problems with mumbling and stammering. However, once the boys can communicate more clearly, the aggressive behaviors that they demonstrate often decrease.

Regulation Disorders and ADHD

As with any child with an additional diagnosis, the child who has both RDSP and ADHD is a more complex child than the child who has only one of these disorders. Not all children with RDSP will have ADHD or vice versa. A subgroup can be defined but they can all be described under the Disruptive Behavior Disorder Not Otherwise Specified (NOS) diagnostic grouping. The usual presentation of ADHD involves problems with attention, impulsivity and hyperactivity. The child with ADHD and RDSP may have more problems because of the aspects of disregulation, temperamental problems, sensory, motor and spatial problems that interact and often compound the problems created by ADHD.

Regulation Disorders and autism

Some children with RDSP mistakenly receive a diagnosis on the autism spectrum. It is easy to see why that would occur. Children who are slow to respond to sensory input often look withdrawn, listless, and only interested in themselves. Infants with a fearful, cautious presentation of RDSP (Type A, Regulation Disorder DC: 0–3R 2005) may show an increased sensitivity to loud noise, or may have tactile defensiveness. DC: 0–3R (2005) describes how these children attempt to escape from a stimulus and sometimes become motorically agitated. Children with an underresponsive pattern, slow motor patterns of limited exploration or restricted play repertoire also demonstrate responses similar to children on the autism spectrum. In addition, children diagnosed with Multisystem Developmental Disorders (MSDD), using the DC: 0–3R system, also show striking similarities to RDSP and ASD. There are very few studies that have looked at these diagnostic dilemmas. In a BCCH clinic study, we found that it was indeed difficult to be accurate about the diagnosis of ASD in young children (Reebye *et al.* 2000). Another study that looked at distinguishing diagnostic boundaries between RDSP and MSDD found that children with RDSP and children with MSDD showed qualitative and quantitative differences in linguistic, behavioral and relational dimensions (Cesari *et al.* 2003).

Greenspan and Weider (1998) reviewed clinical records of 200 children that met the diagnosis of autism or Pervasive Developmental Disorder Not Otherwise Specified (PDD-NOS) (DSM-IV-TR, APA 2000). The charts of each child were followed for at least two years. Children in this study, even with the diagnosis of autism or PDD-NOS, had responses similar to those who are diagnosed with RDSP, with 28 percent demonstrating self-absorption, 19 percent demonstrating hypersensitivity to touch or sound, and 48 percent of the sample having severe motor planning dysfunction.

We have referred elsewhere to our own experience of evolution of diagnostic change in children diagnosed with RDSP (refer to BCCH experience, Reebye 1996; Reebye *et al.* 2000; Reebye and Stalker 2003).

Regulation Disorders and Neonatal Abstinence Disorder

Clinical and scientific information related to the effects on infants born to mothers who abused alcohol during their pregnancy is abundant. Researchers stress evidence of difficulty modulating incoming stimuli and general problem-solving difficulties with children who have prenatal exposure to alcohol (Streissguth and LaDue 1987).

In children exposed to cocaine, neurobehavioral organizational deficits were observed in preclinical (using rat pups) studies (Hume *et al.* 1989) and clinical studies of human fetuses. Disorganized behavioral state in the fetus successfully predicted abnormal newborn behavior. Their findings support the concepts that cocaine exposure disrupts central nervous system development and that fetal assessment of state is predictive of neonatal outcome (Simonik, Robinson and

Smotherman 1993). As there are overlapping constructs of motor and sensory disorganization, one must be aware of these developments, but as yet there is no definite way to make a primary diagnosis of RDSP in children exposed *in utero* to toxic drug substances. Clinical experience tells us that language processing differentiates these children from children with a RDSP diagnosis without any known organic cause. At the time of writing this book, we did not have any empirical findings to support or discard this overlapping symptom presentation.

Regulation Disorders and sleep disorders

DC: 0–3R (2005) describes sleep behavior disorders in a separate category. This category is reserved for two types of sleep disturbances that occur after the age of 12 months.

In the original 0–3 Diagnostic Classification (ZERO TO THREE 1994) there was an emphasis on sleep, eating and elimination patterns within the description of Regulation Disorders. Sleep regulation is one of the major neuroadaptive tasks of early infancy and therefore continues to be relevant to our discussion. However, having sleep disturbance in isolation cannot be included as a criteria for the diagnosis of RDSP.

The available evidence, direction of the DC: 0–3R task force, and clinical experience indicates that sleep disturbance is a common symptom (complaint) but not a necessary condition for the diagnosis of RDSP.

Summary

- RDSPs are multifactorial in origin. Each child has his or her individual sensory, motor, physiological and behavioral processing and organizational patterns and needs. The child with RDSP has more accentuated patterns in some or all of these areas. Diagnosis of RDSP requires that a child exhibit a distinct behavioral pattern, motor difficulties and sensory processing difficulties that are observed over time.

- RDSP in early years can be confused with sleep disorders, Autism Spectrum Disorder and early evolving Attention Deficit Disorder with (or without) hyperactivity. These continue to be commonly considered differential diagnoses.

- The nature of the progression of RDSP is still in the clinical observation domain. There are no long-term research findings that can be uniformly applied. In general, it is believed that RDSP during early childhood might be a harbinger to later difficulties in a child's life. This points to a need for further research and early, preventative interventions for these disorders.

Chapter 2

ASSESSMENT AND DIAGNOSIS
OF REGULATION DISORDERS

When considering each child who may have Regulation Disorders of Sensory Processing (RDSP), the different behaviors and responses can be quantified and graphed in a pie chart. The different proportions of behaviors/responses indicate the areas that affect the child the most – sensory, motor, physiological responses and behavior that includes organization and processing of affect and attention, as well as overall behavioral responses (see Figure 2.1).

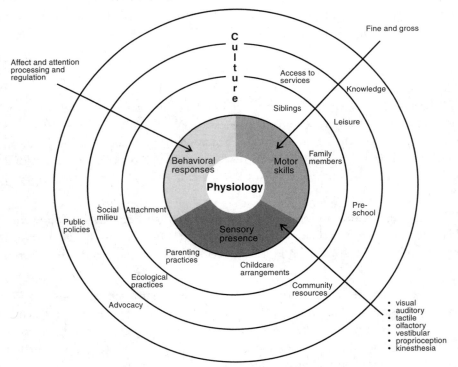

Figure 2.1 Variables affecting Regulation Disorders of Sensory Processing

Context and individuals interacting with the child are additional important variables. Knowledge of the most significant problematic areas and areas of strength of the individual child can help with diagnosis and developing management strategies. After the pie diagram is constructed, diagnosis of RDSP can be aided by the use of specific assessment tools.

Let us consider a child called Thomas and how the pie chart would look during various stages of his development.

As an infant (see Figure 2.2), Thomas demonstrated fussiness and became irritable in high-stimulation situations. He seemed overwhelmed with sensory overloading unless he was held in a horizontal plane rather than the usual vertical position, to lessen visual stimuli. Water temperature was a big issue during baths – a thermometer had to be used to get exactly the right temperature each time (*sensory*). He was late in crawling – preferring to lie on his back and making little effort to initiate rolling or a commando crawl (*motor*). His general behavior appeared withdrawn as a baby – slow to warm up to adults and irritable in high-stimulation situations (*behavior – affect*). He either did not settle or had some difficulty settling when nursing (*physiological*). He had to be in a quiet dark room to be able to attend to breastfeeding for a sustained time. He often needed white noise (such the vacuum cleaner being left on or monotonous music) or to be taken for a car ride to get him to go to sleep. When his mother tried to sing to him to calm him he reacted negatively although he settled for radio music (*sensory, behavior – attention, affect and general behavior*). It was the colic-like behavior, the difficulty in settling and the negative responses to his mother's voice that resulted in a pediatrician sending the family to the infant mental health clinic. He thought there might be a parent–child interaction problem.

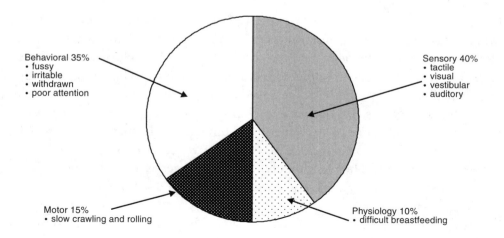

Figure 2.2 Thomas as an infant

In his toddler years (see Figure 2.3), Thomas was difficult to dress and toilet train because of his irritability with new clothes, decreased awareness of wet and dry, and the reaction of screaming and running away in response to the noise of a flushing toilet (*sensory*). He would only eat crunchy foods, avoiding mushy ones, and had a limited number of foods that he would eat (*physiological – eating and sensory*). He continued to be irritable and withdrawn from other children. His parents noted that, in all his early photographs, he looks like an old granny who was in a negative mood (*behavior – affect*). Although now walking, he did not explore his environment and preferred activities, such as looking at books, that meant he was sitting with limited motor responses (*motor*).

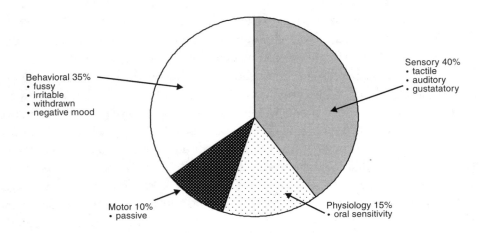

Figure 2.3 Thomas as a toddler

During his preschool years (see Figure 2.4), Thomas continued to be a child who would sit and look at books for long periods of time rather than engage in active play (*motor*). He would hide behind trees and was generally reclusive with children his own age. However, he was affectionate and able to relate to his younger brother and immediate family members. He talked a lot, but the topic was almost exclusively about dinosaurs. He had an encyclopedic knowledge about these animals (*behavior*). Although some of his sensory and physiological issues had lessened (he was toilet trained and had expanded his food preferences) he continued to be sensitive to new clothing. He most frequently could be seen wearing his loose-fitting Batman costume, although his sedentary motor activity did not match his favorite movie character (*sensory*).

As can be seen, Thomas's pie charts changed in proportions of the different domains as we followed him through his early years.

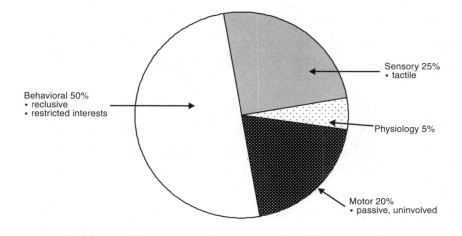

Figure 2.4 Thomas as a preschooler

Discussion

Behavior is dysfunctional if someone (the child, parents or other caregivers) is negatively affected by it. Superficial or singular problems may be important to a particular child; however, it is the *combination of behaviors* that is likely to make the most profound impact on the child's overall functioning. The *cluster of problems* in the following areas – sensory (tactile, olfactory [smell], gustatory [taste], auditory and visual processing, as well as proprioception, kinesthetic and vestibular responses), motor (gross and fine motor), behavioral organization and processing (attention and affect) and overall behavioral responses – and *their persistence over time* makes them of concern. Maladaptive physiological responses (sleeping, eating and/or elimination patterns) may also be present and interact with other problematic behaviors. Each child will have her own individual variations of the behaviors that are represented in each of the sensory, motor, physiological, and behavioral domains. These responses may change from day to day and as the child matures. However, to qualify for a diagnosis of RDSP, a pattern demonstrating sensory difficulties, motor difficulties and a specific behavioral pattern is essential (DC: 0–3R, 2005).

To identify and quantify a child's responses within the pie graph, questions need to be asked about what is being regulated (or not being regulated) in the child's responses within the following areas:

- sensory (tactile, auditory, visual, olfactory, gustatory, kinesthetic, vestibular and proprioceptive senses)

- motor (gross and fine motor)

- behavior (attention and affect)

- physiological (sleep, eating and/or elimination patterns)
- overall behavior.

In addition to identifying the different responses, the following questions need to be considered:

- How much effort does it take for the child to remain in control (e.g. can the child manage play skills with one other child but not a group)?

- What is the role of environment in which the child demonstrates her symptoms of loss or maintenance of control (e.g. is it only in noisy crowded situations, only when she is tired, etc.)?

- Who are the individuals in the child's life and how do they regulate or disregulate the child (e.g. demanding grandparents who expect a quiet orderly child)?

Assessment tools for diagnosing Regulation Disorders

After a pie chart is constructed, diagnosis of RDSP can be aided by the use of standardized assessment tools. Dr. Winnie Dunn has developed three questionnaires that have been standardized for both infants (birth to six months) and toddlers (7 to 36 months) (the *Infant/Toddler Sensory Profile* – Dunn and Daniels 2002) and for children aged 3 to 11 years (the *Sensory Profile* – Dunn 1999, 2005) as well as one for youth and adults. Items explore the areas of sensory processing with children under 36 months and additional aspects of modulation, behavioral and emotional responses for the older children.

Dr. Georgia DeGangi and colleagues developed the *Infant-Toddler Symptom Checklist: Long Version* (DeGangi *et al.* 1995). The checklist is filled in by the parent and considers the areas of self-regulation, attention, movement, listening, language and sound, looking and sight, and attachment – emotional functioning.

Greenspan, DeGangi and Weider (2001) developed *The Functional Emotional Assessment Scale (FEAS) for Infancy and Early Childhood*. This assessment is completed with the primary caregiver playing with the child as well as the examiner facilitating play. The caregiver behaviors in the areas of regulation and interest in the world, attachment, intentional two-way communication, complex sense of self, behavioral organization, representational organization and elaboration and emotional thinking are assessed. Child behaviors are also assessed in the areas of regulation and interest in the world, forming relationships (attachment), intentional two-way communication, complex sense of self, behavioral organization and elaboration, representational capacity and elaboration, and emotional thinking (DeGangi 2000).

Bagnato *et al.* (1999) created *The Temperament and Atypical Behavior Scale (TABS)*. It is a standardized instrument useful for assessing problem behaviors in children between ages one and six years. This is a multicomponent screening and assessment tool based on direct observation and caregiver report used to determine early emerging problems in self-regulation. There is no special training required to administer this assessment.

Types of Regulation Disorders

The Diagnostic Classification ZERO TO THREE – Revised (Diagnostic Category [DC]: 0–3R, 2005) describes three main types of disorders: Hypersensitive (with subtypes Type A Fearful/Cautious and Type B Negative/Defiant), Hyposensitive/Under-responsive, and Sensory Stimulation-Seeking/Impulsive. These categories provide a description of the child as a young baby and toddler. However, this diagnosis can still be valid for children over the age of four. The Revision Task Force concluded that:

> at this stage of our knowledge, DC: 0–3R could neither provide detailed criteria for subtypes of Regulation Disorders of Sensory Processing nor specify the number of criteria needed for diagnosis. Instead, [we] provided criteria in rich descriptive form in the hope that future research will clarify this area. (DC: 0–3R, ZERO TO THREE 2005, p. 12)

This present flexibility makes sense clinically. Many subtypes outlined in the earlier descriptions were seen to be overlapping and changing with rapid developmental changes during infancy and preschool periods. The DC: 0–3R does specify that the diagnosis of Regulation Disorder Sensory Processing (RDSP) includes the presence of the three features of sensory processing difficulties, motor difficulties, and a specific behavioral pattern (see Table 2.1).

Table 2.1 Types of Regulation Disorders of Sensory Processing

Type of problem	Sensory	Motor	Behavior
Hypersensitive Type A (Fearful/Cautious). Aversive reactions to stimuli	Over-reactive to sensory stimuli related to touch, sound, visual, smell, taste, tactile and movement in space, may result in fearfulness, crying or "freezing"	Difficulties with postural control and tone, fine motor coordination, motor planning may result in less exploration and sensory-motor play than expected for the child's age	Excessive caution, inhibition and fearfulness. Infants may demonstrate a restricted range of exploration, limited assertiveness, distress when their routine is changed, and fear and clinginess in new situations. Toddlers and preschoolers may demonstrate excessive fears and worries, shyness to new people, places or objects, distractibility, impulsivity, frequent bouts of irritability and tearfulness, limited ability to self-soothe
Type B (Negative/Defiant). Aversive reactions to stimuli	Sensory reactivity the same as Type A	Motor patterns the same as Type A	Behavioral patterns differ from Type A Avoids or is slow to engage in new experiences, generally aggressive only when provoked. Behaviors include negativistic and controlling behaviors, defiance, preference for repetition, absence or slow rate of change, difficulty in adapting to change, compulsions and perfectionism, avoidance or slow involvement in new experiences or sensory experiences
Hyposensitive/ Under-responsive. Requires high sensory input before child responds	Under-reactive to sound, movement, smell, taste, touch and proprioception Infants show lack of response to sensations and social overtures	Limited explorations and restricted play repertoire. Engages in specific and often repetitive sensory input. Fatigues easily and poor motor planning skills	Quiet and watchful with apparent lack of interest in social activities and interactions, games and objects. Apathetic appearance, tires easily, inattentive, withdrawal from stimuli in the environment

Table 2.1 continued

Type of problem	Sensory	Motor	Behavior
Sensory Stimulation-Seeking/Impulsive. Requires high intensity, frequent and/or sensory input for long periods of time before they respond	Craves high intensity stimuli resulting at times in destructive or safety issues	Need for motor discharge, demonstrates diffuse impulsivity, accident prone without clumsiness	High activity level, seeks constant contact with people and objects, seeks stimulation through deep pressure, recklessness and disorganized behavior. Infants may seek or crave sensory input and stimulation, preschoolers may appear excitable, aggressive, intrusive, daring and reckless, preoccupied with aggressive themes in play

Summary

- A comprehensive history from parents/caregivers and a multidisciplinary team assessment is the core of the diagnostic procedures involved in RDSP. As well, various assessment tools to measure sensory integration difficulties and social–emotional development of the child are available. The Diagnostic Classification ZERO TO THREE – Revised (DC: 0–3R, 2005) describes three main types of RDSP:

  1. Hypersensitive (with subtypes Type A Fearful/Cautious and Type B Negative/Defiant)

  2. Hyposensitive/Under-responsive

  3. Sensory Stimulation-Seeking/Impulsive.

- The diagnosis of RDSP includes the presence of the three features of sensory processing difficulties, motor difficulties, and a specific behavioral pattern.

Chapter 3

THE DEVELOPMENT OF REGULATION DURING INFANCY, TODDLER, PRESCHOOL AND EARLY SCHOOL YEARS

The development of a baby's brain

Whether responding to the needs of an adult, child or infant, it is our brain that mediates and interprets all of the information that is presented to us.

The functions of the various areas of the brain develop in discrete stages. Babies learn to use their nervous system even during their intrauterine life. Brain development commences soon after conception and continues postnatally. Awareness of this factor is important because it points to the significance of postnatal experiences on the baby's developing brain. This postnatal development is rapid until age two to three years but there is evidence to support that it continues into adolescence (Huttenlocher 1994). It is possible to now record fetal neurobehavioral stages described as occurring after 36 weeks. The fetal behavioral state parameters are eye movements, body movements and fetal heart rate (Dipietro 2001).

The third trimester to two years of age is seen as a critical period in brain development since the brain is open to experiential suggestions. These experiences can be positive or negative with the baby's susceptibility determined by genetic potential. The baby's brain is endowed with billions of neurons at birth, but the postnatal experiences can "prune" (delete) or enhance/accelerate synapse formation. Thus, neurodevelopmental aspects of infant regulation capacities are both genetically and environmentally interactive and influence self-organization of the developing brain (Schore 1994).

Recognition of the importance of early positive nurturing experiences for the infant cannot be minimized (see Figure 3.1). The impact of facilitating central brain circuitry for organization and modulation capacities in the experience-dependent postnatal brain has to be respected.

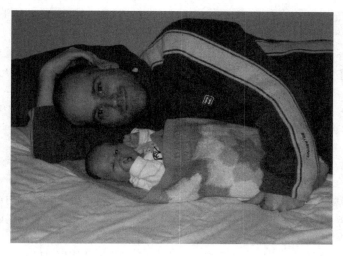

Figure 3.1 Nurturing moments

Regulation Disorders in infants

A variety of "irregularities" are seen within normal infants up to the age of 12 months. These may be in the areas of sleep disturbances, digestion and self-calming abilities. However, for most children these difficulties resolve with minimal or no intervention.

Fussy babies have always existed. In one study, up to 29 percent of infants suffered from excessive crying (James-Roberts 1991; James-Roberts and Halil 1991). Other studies indicated 15–25 percent had sleep problems (Kirjavainen *et al.* 2001; Richman 1981) and 36 percent had feeding problems (Forsyth and Canny 1991) in otherwise healthy infants. So although these irritable, disregulated babies have always existed, what is new is our understanding of them and the development of a diagnostic construct which tries to encompass the sensory, motor and behavioral processing difficulties of these infants and children.

The infants that persist with difficulties mentioned above are now grouped under the diagnostic description of Regulation Disorders of Sensory Processing (RDSP).

The question has often been asked how this construct is different from variations in temperament seen in individual babies and children. Temperament is seen
as a collection of attributes unique to each child (see Chess and Thomas 1996; Fox
2004 for detailed information) while Regulation Disorders can be altered with
intervention (DeGangi *et al.* 1996; Fox 2004; Richman 1981). The usual procedure
to assess temperament is through parental reports and laboratory-based assessments (Buss and Goldsmith 1998).

Diagnosis of RDSP requires a multidisciplinary approach with a team of child
psychiatrist, psychologist, occupational therapist, and speech and language therapist utilizing multiple assessment tools and methods.

There are significant changes during early infancy as babies reorganize their
perceptions of themselves and others. Stern (1985, p. 8) noted, "At each of these
major shifts, infants create a forceful impression that major changes have occurred
in their subjective experience of self and other." These biobehavioral shifts are
described as occurring at 2–3 months, 9–12 months and 15–18 months of age.
The first shift is when biological rhythmicity is at risk. The second biobehavioral
shift signifies organization within the infant's self and development of an inner
world. During this time, sleep problems and separation anxiety can become overwhelming. The third shift is marked by the toddler wanting to achieve independence and autonomy, but also seeking contact with the important caregivers in his
life. This negotiation of needs contributes to overall regulation of impulses, and
abilities to be independent and interdependent.

The regulation learning tasks of infancy

Think about a mother who, through normal delivery, produces a beautiful healthy
baby. This baby within a few hours is facing a completely new world of strangers,
noise and stimuli. To cope with this, the child may completely ignore the stimuli, or
show an altered state of regulation varying from alert to a drowsy state or sleep.
Alternately the child may respond by excessive crying or agitation.

Infants are intrinsically different from older toddlers and children. They differ
in their physical abilities, temperament, and ability to regulate their responses to
both the outside world and their inner world. During the first year, mastery over
sensory functions is the major victory in learning self-regulation. It is important
for adaptation to the environment and to establish homeostasis (predictability and
stability of responses).

This initial task of infancy – of maintaining internal homeostasis – also
requires infants to explore their immediate environment. They learn new tasks and
respond to the ambience established by their caretaker, all the while without losing

previously learned functions. In addition, family affect and behavioral codes have to be learned and assimilated.

Infants can use their touch, vision, and voice to regulate their responses to these stimuli. Some manage better than others, but eventually all children learn to control the stimuli in some way. Babies and toddlers with RDSP often develop unique and disregulated responses in an attempt to cope.

Scaffolding (an adult providing support and direction) to help the baby regulate is important so the infant can increase attention and self-regulation. The infant cannot integrate these aspects without the help of a nurturing caregiver. The caregiver needs to match the infant's signals through visual gestures, tactile and verbal responses (see Figure 3.2). For new parents, these subtle clues are often difficult to decipher in a normally responding baby, and doubly so in a baby with RDSP.

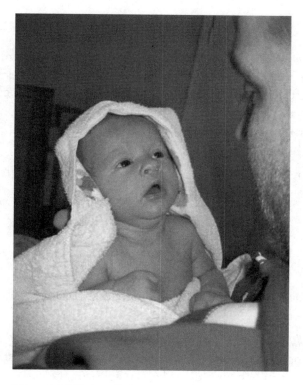

Figure 3.2 Mind reading

Behavioral and sensory responses in the infant with Regulation Disorders

In infants with RDSP, the following responses seem most evident as being poorly organized.

Sensory

The infant may demonstrate under- or over-reactivity to odors and to bright lights or visual images that are new or unique. Tactile defensiveness may be demonstrated by over-reactivity to dressing, bathing, cutting nails, cutting hair or oral hypersensitivity where there is avoidance of certain textured food. This may be accompanied by oral motor difficulties with chewing and swallowing. Under- or over-reactivity to touch and pain, temperature and loud noises or high-pitched sounds may be experienced.

Motor

- *Gross motor activity*: Even as a small infant, motor disorganization with jerky and constant movement may be observed. At different times, poorly differentiated, sparse or limp movements may occur. As the infant begins to sit and stand, gravitational insecurity, poor muscle tone and decreased muscle instability may be demonstrated.

- *Fine motor activity*: Qualitative deficits may be seen in motor planning skills, motor modulation of motor movements and fine motor skills related to the development of refined grasp and pincer grip.

Physiological

The infant may demonstrate irregular breathing, hiccups, gagging, and startle easily.

- *Elimination difficulties*: Bowel and elimination patterns may be inconsistent.

- *Sleeping difficulties*: The infant may have problems settling, difficulty developing progressively longer periods of sleep and restless sleeping habits. A sleep behavior disorder is diagnosed if sleep disturbance continues to occur after age 12 months.

- *Feeding difficulties*: The child may have oral sensitivities resulting in difficulty nursing, irritability or disinterest when nursing and be slow to accept solids.

Behavioral processing and organization

- *Perceptual processing.* The infant may have perceptual problems in auditory and visual areas and qualitative deficits in visual spatial processing capacities, although these deficits are difficult to identify in the young infant.

- *Attention organization.* The infant may appear to have "driven" behaviors with an inability to settle and limited capacity to attend and focus for an age-appropriate time.

- *Affect organization.* The infant's range of affect may shift rapidly from being calm to screaming frantically.

Overall behavioral organization

The beginnings of aggressive or impulsive behaviors may emerge with persistent crying, irritability and lack of attention.

Language

Qualitative deficits in articulation capacity may be heard as the infant begins to make initial sounds and sound patterns.

The regulation learning tasks during the toddler years

During the toddler years, from about one to three years of age, children are beginning to interact with other people beyond their immediate family members, to become mobile and explore their world, to learn to speak and interact both by asking questions and giving information, and to begin to identify themselves as individuals.

Regulation tasks during this age are to begin to participate in managing their responses in all of the areas of sensory, motor, physiological, organization and processing and behavioral responses. Much of the regulation is still initiated and modulated by the parent(s)/caregiver but the child is expected to at least be aware of the adult's intervention and responsive to it.

Behavioral and sensory responses in the toddler with Regulation Disorders

In toddlers with RDSP, the following responses seem most evident as being poorly organized.

Sensory

Continued or apparent increased or decreased sensitivity in areas of visual, auditory, tactile, oral, olfactory and gustatory senses, and increased or decreased pain and temperature awareness may occur. Because the child is now becoming mobile, these sensitivities or lack (e.g. temperature awareness) may lead to safety issues.

Motor

- *Gross motor activity*: Motor coordination problems may become more apparent with walking occurring later than usual and observance of unsteady gait or balance. The child may have constant movement or limited movement and demonstrate poor muscle tone, postural insecurity or limited range in types of motor movements.

- *Fine motor activity*: Problems with fine motor modulation and planning skills become more apparent as the child is expected to play with more sophisticated toys that require taking apart, placement, and movement. As well, more refined pincer grip and flexible hand and wrist movement may be limited and this affects both self-care and pre-academic learning tasks.

Physiological

- *Elimination difficulties*: The introduction of toilet-training routines may result in the toddler becoming resistant or indifferent.

- *Sleeping difficulties*: The toddler may have difficulty falling and staying asleep, and experience night terrors and dreams.

- *Feeding difficulties*: The toddler may make selective choices of food, picking specific textures, colors and/or tastes that limit experiencing a variety of foods.

Behavioral processing and organization

- *Perceptual processing*: Perceptual problems may be more obvious in auditory and visual areas because language responses are expected and toys and interactions require more awareness of visual clues and spatial awareness.

- *Attention organization*: Following directions, remembering information, and attending to clues in the environment become an expectation for the child to learn and participate within the family and with others. Intense focus on small details may become more apparent, or the child may be inattentive and overly active.

- *Affect organization*: At this age, the child is more able to express his feelings and respond by one or more words but often has extreme responses that do not match the situation. The child is difficult to settle when upset and does not necessarily respond to soothing by an adult.

Overall behavioral organization

Aggressive or impulsive behaviors may increase in response to the child's sensory reactions or if the child is thwarted in doing his perseverative behaviors. Behavioral issues may emerge as the child reacts, seeks out and/or resists involvement in the areas of heightened or lowered sensitivity. Disorganized behaviors in high-stimulation family or community situations may occur.

Language

Language acquisition is a complex task that can easily be affected by processing difficulties or external influences. For example, a child with RDSP who feels pressured to perform for caregivers would be more at a disadvantage in attaining complex language. Qualitative deficits in articulation capacity become more apparent as an expectation to speak clearly, learn the family language and respond in conversations and to directions become more frequent.

The regulation learning tasks during the preschool and early school years

The learning tasks for children aged four to six in preschool and early school years become increasingly complicated as the children are expected to respond to complex institutional and societal rules as well as attain academic skills. On a daily basis, their world extends beyond the nuclear family and accommodation to their unique needs may no longer occur.

In all areas of regulation, the child is expected to have more autonomy in managing and responding to sensory, motor, physiological, processing and organization and behavioral needs.

Behavioral and sensory responses in the preschool and early school-age child with Regulation Disorders

In preschool and the early school-age child with RDSP, the following responses seem most evident as being poorly organized.

Sensory

Mild to extreme reactions to sight, sound, smell and taste may interfere with attaining a variety of experiences in the school, home and community settings.

Motor

- *Gross motor activity*: Awkward movements and slower speed (or fast erratic and unsafe speeds), and decreased ability, all present safety concerns when participating in age-appropriate physical activities. As well, social isolation may begin as other children reject the child who lacks coordination from their play groups.

- *Fine motor activity*: The child may experience difficulty in participating in age-appropriate self-care, printing, games and craft activities.

Physiological

- *Elimination difficulties*: Delayed toilet training, night wetting may occur.

- *Sleeping difficulties*: Sleeping irregularities may continue during this age. The adaptation required for a child to respond to early daycare hours or extended daycare as parents return to work and disruption of an established naptime may result in the child presenting as irritable and inattentive.

- *Feeding difficulties*: Children at preschool and school are expected to be fairly independent in chewing, swallowing, and tolerating a wide variety of tastes, textures and smells. In the school environment, if a child limits his intake to a small variety of food it becomes more obvious and limits the child's overall experiences. Additional physiological responses often seen at this age (but which are age inappropriate) are the startle reactions to loud noises, tactile sensitivity, and shuddering as people approach them.

Behavioral processing and organization

- *Perceptual processing:* Perceptual problems in auditory and visual areas may affect academic and social responses. Qualitative deficits in visual spatial processing capacities may affect learning of academic materials and limit involvement in active games.

- *Attention organization:* Inability to attend to a task or perseveration on small details interferes with completion of academic work and social interactions.

- *Affect organization:* Over- or under-reactivity to emotional events as well as difficulty interpreting more complex emotional cues may occur and affect social relationships.

Overall behavioral organization

Responses involving aggressive or impulsive behaviors may alienate the child from peers and a labeling process as a "disturbed" child may begin. The quiet, withdrawn, low-energy child is not included in play activities or noticed for academic tasks requiring initiation.

Language

Language for social and academic activities may lack sophistication in both understanding of input and expressive areas. Written expression also becomes an expectation as part of language skills and may lack descriptive and expanded use of language. Difficulties in sequencing, and understanding subtleties and meaning of language, may be observed.

Summary

- During the first year of life, mastery over sensory functions is the major self-regulation learning task and important for adaptation to the environment and to establish predictability and stability of responses.

- Toddlers need to begin to participate in managing their responses in all of the areas of sensory, motor, physiological, organization, processing and behavioral responses. During preschool and early school years, the child is expected to have more autonomy in managing sensory, behavioral and motor tasks.

- Difficulty in positive and progressive development in the areas of sensory, motor and behavioral management affects emotional, self-care, play and academic skills.

Chapter 4

THERAPEUTIC APPROACHES FOR THE CHILD WITH REGULATION DISORDERS

Treatment planning should not be confined to input by professionals alone. Both parents and professionals need to understand the responses of the child within the domains of sensory, motor, physiological, and behavioral responses. By developing and referring to a "pie" diagram to understand the proportion or importance given to each of these areas for each specific child, the types of treatment that may best suit the child can be decided.

Let us consider Michael, the three-and-a-half-year-old son of Mr. and Mrs. Doe. Michael was always a fussy infant. However, his parents, being first-time parents, did not realize that his frequent waking up at night, insisting on only drinking bottled milk at a particular temperature and screaming when he was brought to noisy shopping malls was different than other children of his age. Admirably, they coped with all of the distress during the first year. Just when it seemed the family and Michael were beginning to settle down, the family had to relocate to a town where the weather in winter was severe. Michael could not tolerate having his head covered, mittens on his hands, or thick socks and constantly cried and fussed when dressed for the outdoors. His tactile sensitivity was so extreme that his parents could only dress him in soft flannels, whatever the season. At home, he was happiest when he could just wear his underpants, and always felt very "hot." He did not like the restraint of car seats and did not allow his mother to shampoo his hair.

Dinnertime brought more woes to the family. Michael insisted on eating dry cereal and anything mushy was instantly rejected. He liked crunchy vegetables and meat so at least he could be well nourished. He had a high activity level and seldom sat still for family meals. The parents tried to accommodate his preferences, to maintain family peace if for no other reason.

What brought them for consultation at the infant mental health clinic was an incident where his mother had to be hospitalized for minor surgery and he was left in the care of his mother's girlfriend. Michael howled, screamed and, when he cried, he sweated a lot on his forehead. As usual, he did not want to wear clothes. When invited by other children to play indoor games, he refused to play at first. When he finally joined them, he hugged one of the children of his age so tightly that the child started crying, almost suffocated, and refused to play with him. This incident was seen by the adults present as an act of aggression and Michael's parents decided to bring him for consultation. Plotting a pie diagram can help to understand Michael's difficulties better (see Figure 4.1).

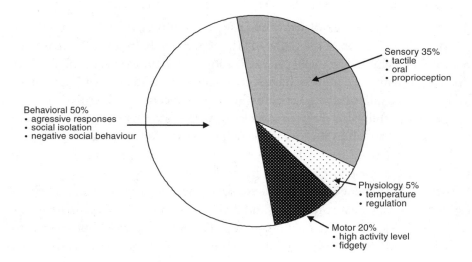

Figure 4.1 Regulation Disorders experienced by Michael

By deciding what domains represent the most pressing concerns, referral can be made to the different types of professionals who might be able to help this family.

In this case, sensory responses appear the most pressing.

- *Sensory*: Auditory (noisy malls), oral (crunchy food preference), tactile (prefers to not wear clothes, resistant to restraints such as car seat, resistant to hair washing), proprioceptive (seeking deep hugs). An occupational therapist could use sensory integration approaches to help lessen the intensity of sensory responses and make recommendations to home and school of adaptations and modifications that could help Michael to improve his function in these settings.

- *Motor*: High activity level and fidgety behaviors. A psychiatrist could help with behavior management strategies for Michael and his parents and might consider if medication was needed.

- *Physiological*: Sweating when upset. A psychiatrist could discuss this response with the parents to help them understand its origins and how to manage the response.

- *Behavioral*: Screaming, upset, preferred to play alone, striking out. Multidisciplinary team members can consult together and present a cohesive management plan possibly involving instruction in behavioral modification and reward systems, child-centered play, response to sensory needs and methods to encourage social interactions.

There is a need to look at each of the domains and the sub-categories within them, and the overall behavior responses of the child to help define treatment approaches. Some children do well on medication; some do worse. Some families are helped by learning general behavior management strategies; other families already have these skills and need specific help with specific problem areas.

The age of the child also dictates some approaches. For instance, when a child is young it is more difficult to sort out if the behaviors are Attention Deficit Hyperactivity Disorder (ADHD) or Regulation Disorders of Sensory Processing (RDSP) so fine tuning of interventions may take longer.

For Michael, it can be seen that he has sensory, physiological, motor and behavioral responses that all create problems, and that his responses to his sensory needs often lead to behaviors that are misinterpreted. The best help would be to start to assess the degree of his sensory regulation issues with the occupational therapist taking the lead in a multidisciplinary assessment and treatment decision-making process.

There is a need to consider who is being regulated when a treatment plan is developed. When the children are attending preschool, the child, family, school, community and clinicians need to consider their own regulation of their responses so they can provide a safe and supportive environment for the child. This ability of the adults who are involved with the child, to regulate their own behaviors and sensory responses, will lead to effective regulation of the child's environment. This self-regulation develops from knowledge about the condition, a positive relationship with the child, an ability to be consistent, skills in analyzing the precursors and causes of the child's disregulated behaviors, and access to adult support systems for the caregivers. Maintaining a positive relationship with the child throughout her childhood is the most important factor.

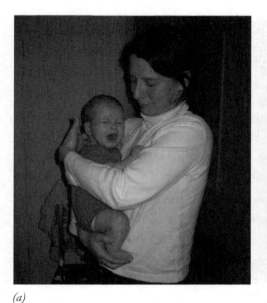
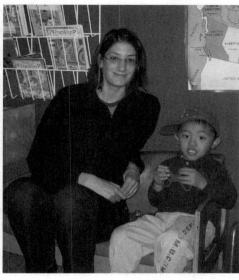

(a)   *(b)*

Figures 4.2a and b Early regulators

Other adults including educators and health professionals can help assist the child to learn to regulate herself (see Figures 4.2a and b). The same potential helpers can also inadvertently disregulate the child by anxious, frustrated or angry responses to both parents and their child.

As each child matures and enters school and community activities, all adults will need to help the children to learn strategies to manage their own emotional and sensory responses. However, adults will also need to continue to help adapt or modify the environment and to advocate for each child within systems (educational, medical, community) so they can participate in age-appropriate activities, while they learn and practice these strategies.

Therapeutic approaches

Many therapeutic approaches are prescribed to help children with RDSP. This is because the infants, toddlers and children with RDSP are not a homogeneous group and thus require individual and varied approaches.

The approaches that have claimed modest success are the following:

- *Infant–parent psychotherapy* is an approach that tries to help parents to understand their caregiving patterns by working on the parents' emotional liabilities as they affect their parenting abilities. This approach aims to improve the fit between the infant and the caregiver by also understanding infant characteristics (Lieberman and Pawl 1993).

- *Parent–infant interaction guidance* has as a primary goal, to assist the families to make their parenting enjoyable and allow parents to understand their child's behavior and development through play experiences. A working alliance with families involved in therapy is the most important principle (McDonough 1995).

- *Infant-led guidance using intuitive approaches* is an approach that makes use of infant cues and behavior to help the parents to respond appropriately to the direct and indirect cues given by their baby. It has been used with infants with persistent crying (Papousek 2000, 2005).

- *Short-term dynamic psychotherapy* for infants and their parents focuses on the core conflict that is upsetting the parent–child relationship and is practiced as brief therapy (Cramer 1976; Papousek 2000, 2005).

- *Sensory integration therapy* is an approach that helps parents to understand and participate in encouraging the child to develop appropriate responses or learn coping strategies to aversive sensory input or to increase responsiveness to sensory input (Ayers 1994; Ottenbacher 1982; Papousek 2000, 2005).

- *Medication* is appropriate for some children who are distressed over a long period of time because of their inability to regulate their sensory system, their emotions or physiological responses. Medication can help the child to attend and regulate her responses better. This does not mean that the child will be on medications for a lifetime, but it may help mediate responses when they are most extreme.

Treatment principles

A number of considerations should be made when recommending or selecting treatment approaches.

Treatment should be based on information gained from the parents and a thorough assessment of all areas of the child's development. An understanding needs to be developed of the general coping methods of the family, parenting approaches and attachment styles of the parents. As well, awareness needs to be attained of parental factors that may contribute to the situation – such as attributions given to the child's behavior, projections, and distortions about the situation and child that the parents may have developed.

An understanding of the complex interplay between sensory, motor, physiological, and behavioral responses within the individual child needs to be developed.

Treatment should be specific to the unique needs of the individual child and her family.

Multidisciplinary approaches help develop a more diverse understanding of the symptoms of children with RDSP and have also been seen as more effective when families have multiple stressors, e.g. for children with RDSP who are living in stressful environments (Zeanah and Larrieu 1998).

Multidisciplinary teams can include a psychiatrist or psychologist providing guidance and support for the parents, an occupational therapist working with the parents to assess and treat sensory and motor issues, a speech and language pathologist helping the child if there are language-processing issues, the family receiving support in their home from a community health nurse, as well as identification of appropriate daycare, respite care or supported childcare resources by any of the team members.

Initiating treatment

The diagnosis and treatment plan should be developed with the family and a multidisciplinary team working together. Treatment goals should reflect what is realistically remediable considering the resources of the child, parent and community. The child's strengths need to be defined and encouraged. Treatment staff need to maintain awareness of the pitfalls of focusing on the child's weaknesses when developing a treatment plan. Medication education is an important part of parental education if this is a treatment recommended for the child. This involves clearly explaining the mechanism of action of the medications and their possible side effects to the parents (Kutcher 1997; Zeanah and Larrieu 1998).

Support and bridging information should be used to foster higher developmental levels for the child and family. Both parents and therapists must challenge the child and help them to function at the highest level that they can attain. In each area of treatment, progress will not be a fast sequence of "a to b" but will more likely be step by step, "1a, 1b, 2a, 2b," etc. and parents and therapists will need patience.

The helping professional team

For effective assessment, diagnosis and treatment of infants and children with RDSP a team of an infant psychiatrist, occupational therapist, speech and language pathologist, and developmental psychologist is essential. Each of these professionals brings an expertise that can help with both assessment, diagnosis and treatment suggestions.

- An *infant psychiatrist* provides an overall assessment, with a specific focus on a relational and socio-emotional assessment. They establish grounds for the diagnosis and most importantly are able to rule out sleep disorders and feeding disorders in isolation as well as other developmental difficulties (e.g. autism) and disorders exhibited as self-regulation difficulties.

- An *occupational therapist* provides a focused assessment of sensory integration, motor, perceptual and early cognitive skills, as well as self-help activities of daily living, social interactions and play skills.

- A *developmental psychologist* provides an assessment of the child's overall cognitive skills and defines difficulties that may be linked with a communication deficit.

- A *speech and language pathologist* provides assessments of expressive and receptive language and communication deficits as well as social pragmatic language.

It is essential that *all* early childhood clinicians be able to identify RDSP. However, a firm diagnosis of this condition and ensuing recommendations is best done within a multidisciplinary team approach.

A child-centered treatment approach: from restricted to rich fantasy play

Although all of the treatment approaches must be child-centered, some of the children need a more intensive approach to respond to their limited capacity to regulate their environment. Some children with RDSP may demonstrate restricted fantasy, perseveration and over-focusing and can benefit from approaches such as the DIR (**D**evelopmental level, **I**ndividual differences, **R**elationship based) approach described by Dr. Weider and Dr. Greenspan (Greenspan and Weider 1998; Weider and Greenspan 2003).

It is quite common to see children within a mental health clinic who will not play with anything but Lego or only read spaceship books. As compared with children with Autism Spectrum Disorder (ASD), the children with RDSP do have a richer fantasy imagination. Mastery over a specific type of play keeps them motivated, and then, if sensory responses and sometimes over-regulation (which also can contribute to RDSP) are present, these potentially quite capable children are caught in a perseverative pattern.

Techniques used to encourage development of a symbolic world should be selected to promote appropriate growth of developmental skills and should respect the child's sensory reactivity, processing and motor planning skills while helping the child to develop more flexible mental thought processes.

Within the play, trusting relationships are encouraged and an environment of safety, protection, and security is developed.

Throughout the child's waking hours there needs to be constructed opportunities to play with the child. Focusing on what the child is doing in her play and following the child's cues is essential. It is not as easy as it may seem to keep on the play track and only focus and follow a child's direction. However, this is one of the major essential therapeutic guidelines described in the DIR model. Throughout this model, it is suggested that symbolic meaning be assigned to objects and gestures to encourage expansion of ideas and build upon the often concrete play with more imaginative play. This is giving a jump-start to the child who might be stuck with one idea. Later, space, time and nurturance will help the child to learn it is acceptable to make mistakes. Parents will continue to need to help bridge the child's thinking, and to assign emotional content to the play themes.

Some examples of interactions outlined by Dr. Weider and Dr. Greenspan in their Floor Time approach are summarized below. More extensive explanation and instructions of the Floor Time approach are provided in their book *The Child With Special Needs: Encouraging Intellectual and Emotional Growth* (Greenspan and Weider 1998). Explore if there are any psychologists, occupational therapists or other qualified professionals in your community to help you learn the Floor Time approaches.

- Focus on what the child is doing in her play – do not try to teach the child how to do the task better.

- Follow the child's lead – but also elaborate on her intentions and play. Discuss what it appears the child is doing – check it out with the child if that is what she meant.

- Give cues to actions and comment on choices and actions – "I see that you had the teddy upset all his food!"

- Convert real situations into pretend – "The children are sitting at the table and all of a sudden the table turned into a flying carpet!"

- Assign symbolic meaning to objects and gestures. "The dolly is sitting on a very special chair. When she is on the chair she is the one to give orders."

- Match or vary your tone with the child's tone of voice to get the child to attend to your input or questions.

- Use props (puppets and toy action figures) and then substitute one prop for another to help develop flexibility and maintain attention.

- Talk to familiar toy figures such as Mickey Mouse or Barney to model conversations. Many children have seen interactive conversations happening with these characters on television.

- For older children, identify abstract themes that are happening during the play sessions "I think all the animals were feeling sad today – next day they may feel differently."

(Adapted from Weider, S. (1997) "Creating connections: intervention guidelines for increasing interaction with children with Multisystem Developmental Disorder (MSDD)," *Zero to Three Journal*, April/May, 1–27. Copyright © ZERO TO THREE 1997. Reprinted with kind permission.)

Summary

- Treatment approaches for children with RDSP should be developed with the family and multidisciplinary team working in a collaborative fashion.

- Both the treatment approach(es) selected and the development of goals need to consider the resources of the child, parent and community.

Possible treatments include infant–parent psychotherapy, parent–infant interaction guidance, and infant-led guidance using intuitive approaches, short-term dynamic psychotherapy, sensory integration therapy, and medication. Children with restricted fantasy, perseveration and over-focusing may benefit from approaches such as Floor Time.

Part Two

MANAGING REGULATION DISORDERS

Chapter 5

SENSORY RESPONSES

The development of sensory responses

When babies are born, they already have a sensory response system. They are alert to some stimuli, and do not respond to others. They cry when hungry or wet, and settle when fed, comforted and are dry. A major developmental task for newborn infants is to expand and modulate their responses to the various senses in an integrated fashion, so they can self-soothe or alert to stimuli and engage in interactions and learning (see Figures 5.1a and b).

During the first two years of life, the toddler gradually learns to regulate his world by attending, selecting responses to the stimuli, and organizing information to guide thought, action and coordinated movements. Toddlers develop language to help modulate both sensory and verbal contact with the world, and they increase their mobility, resulting in new learning experiences.

During preschool years, children refine coordination skills in the areas of fine motor (e.g. cutting, pencil, dressing skills) and gross motor (e.g. jumping, running, skipping, ball skills), and increase their capacity to use language for interactions, learning and to modify their own and others' responses to sensory input.

School-age children need to have highly refined and integrated behavioral, sensory and processing skills to respond to the demands and structure of a busy classroom and community activities. Even the most basic school work requires a combination of perceptual skills, fine motor skills and auditory, visual and cognitive processing and intermittent or ongoing input from other senses. There is also an expectation for development of more complex abstract thinking processes to extend learning beyond concrete representation of what is seen, felt or heard. Community activities require refined gross and fine motor skills, social skills and behavior self-management.

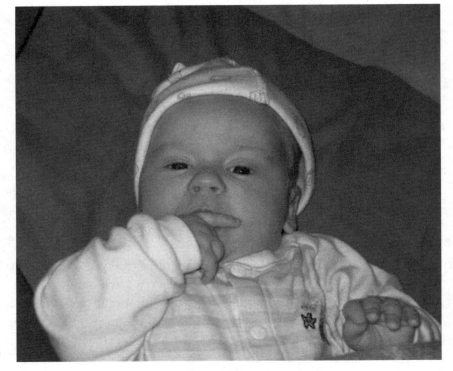

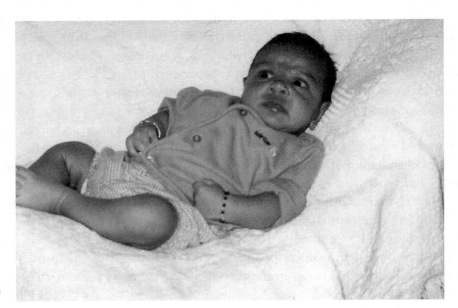

Figures 5.1and b A major developmental task for a newborn infant is to self-soothe

What is sensory integration?

Sensory integration is the neurological processes by which the brain takes in, sorts, regulates and then organizes and interprets our sensory experiences. If there are problems with sensory regulation, a person may be over- or under-sensitive to ordinary stimulation. If there are problems with sensory processing, then organization and interpretation of the information may be difficult.

At a basic level, our sensory systems provide us with input for survival. Our senses consist of tactile (touch sensations), auditory (hearing), visual (seeing), gustatory (taste) and olfactory (smell) senses. There are also internal senses that give us information about the position and movement of our body. These senses are vestibular (responses to information about gravity and movement and position in space), proprioception (unconscious responses to information about the position of body parts and their movement gained through muscles and joint sensation) and kinesthetic (our conscious awareness of how our body is moving). We are generally unaware of these three internal senses and of the sensory system that regulates physiological responses such as hunger, temperature, and attention. Awareness occurs only when something is not going well, e.g. balance does not occur when we need it to perform a movement task.

At a more complex level our senses simultaneously process multiple inputs to help us to attend, learn from and respond appropriately to the environment and the people within it.

What is sensory-integrative dysfunction?

Children may be hypersensitive (over-reacting) or hyposensitive (under-reacting) to sensory input. Depending on the child's own unique responses, the situation, level of fatigue, hunger or health, the child's responses can fluctuate and result in hypersensitivity for some senses and hyposensitivity for others.

For children who have severe sensory responses (with hypersensitive or hyposensitive/under-responsive or sensory stimulation-seeking/impulsive responses), assessment and treatment by an occupational therapist trained in sensory integration is recommended. Severity can be measured by the amount of interference in daily activities the lowered and/or heightened sensory responses create. If the child has difficulty participating successfully in the activities that their peers enjoy and complete, if they are over- or under-reactive to common events in their environment, then clearly defining their sensory and learning profile and developing strategies to address their needs is important (Ayers 1994; Aquilla 2000; Yack, Sutton and Aquilla 2002).

On the following pages we will describe a variety of senses and present questions that an educator, clinician or parent should ask to see if the child taught, assessed or parented is demonstrating sensitivities in this area. Remember – it is *patterns of sensitivities, frequency of the reactions* and *severity of the problem* rather than an intermittent or one-time event that makes the responses noteworthy.

Everyone has some mild sensitivities in a variety of areas (e.g. reactions to bright flashing strobe lights, fingernails scratching on a chalkboard, etc.) so it is important to differentiate when the problem is significant.

The strategies suggested in this book are intended to help develop a thought process and problem-solving strategies to lead to possible approaches to manage the challenges presented by a child with Regulation Disorders of Sensory Processing (RDSP). Additional suggestions can be found in the books listed in the Resources section or in books focused on treatment strategies for children with Asperger's Syndrome or High Functioning Autism and for children with Attention Deficit Disorder.

An effective first step in developing management strategies for any problem presented by a child with Regulation Disorders can be to use the same sequence that we teach children for solving problems.

- Define the problem – how did the child react, what was the environment, what happened preceding, during and after the behaviour, what sensory input was happening?

- Think of at least three approaches that might help to solve the problem.

- Choose the approach that will best match the child's sensory, motor, behavioral and physiological needs.

- Try the chosen approach.

- If it is not effective, analyze why it didn't work and try one of the other possible approaches.

With this approach, and by selection of strategies that increase positive sensory and behavioral responsiveness, the child can be helped to learn self-regulation.

Visual sensitivities

Visual sensation is a response to sight and light. Some children with RDSP are fascinated by light and shadow; others find bright lights or colors very aversive. They may be unusually sensitive, or unresponsive to other aspects of sight and light.

Questions to consider

1. Does visual stimuli interfere with the child's attention or increase discomfort and arousal to a distressing level? Consider each stimulus separately to grade the events and define the type of interference.

2. Does the child have problems linking sights and sounds – where the sound is coming from, or to what visual object the sound is attached?

3. Does the child have difficulty linking sight and touch, sight and smell, sight and movement? Does multisensory stimulation increase distress levels?

4. Does the child hesitate when moving down from a curb or jumping off objects? These problems may indicate difficulties with binocular vision (depth perception) or responses to vestibular stimulation (movement and gravity information).

5. Can the child (school-age) match and sort objects, clothes, alphabet letters?

6. Does the child have difficulty finding clothes or toys in a box, matching objects, or placing things in designated areas? These problems may indicate perceptual problems (e.g. figure ground, form constancy, spatial relations).

7. Does the child miss visual social detail – the feelings expressed on others' faces and the body language? Problems in this area may result in impaired social skills.

8. If the child is relaxed, can he cope with the visual stimuli?

9. Can the child independently disengage from the visual stimuli?

10. Is the child unaware or disinterested in looking at objects, or not alert to colorful visual occurrences?

11. Does the child prefer a darkened room or a room with no bright lights?

12. Does the child become over-excited when in a visually stimulating environment?

13. Is the child constantly alert to all visual detail?

14. Does the child create and/or look intensely at moving objects such as his own flapping hands or whirling fans, dripping water or blinking lights?

15. Does the child seek stimuli by looking carefully at the detail of objects or books for long periods of time?

16. Is visual memory (the ability to retain visually perceived experiences) a strength for the child?

Management strategies

Natural lighting or indirect lighting used in areas where the child must concentrate on tasks may help. Teach children to look away or cover their eyes if there is a bright light or color that bothers them (see Figures 5.2a and b). However, this avoidance strategy must be accompanied by talk about safety aspects, e.g. do not cover your eyes when walking across the street.

A great deal of learning occurs through our visual senses. If children are overwhelmed by visual detail they may find it hard to attend to information presented in a visual manner. When children need to attend, let them close their eyes while they listen. Develop a hand signal to alert children to redirect their visual focus to a task. If they need to observe, isolate the item/activity so it is not surrounded by a lot of extra visual information.

A homework/play space that is free from visual distractions, such as open storage shelves and busy wallpaper, will help the child to attend to the task at hand. Use boxes with lids and containers that can slide into shelving for toys.

To increase efficiency in visual tasks, help the child learn to systematically scan a picture to gain details. Encourage use of language to describe visual details the child needs to retain.

Develop a multisensory approach to learning at home and school and play games in which the child can talk about just what they feel or hear or smell. Help them to experience and understand that all the senses help us to learn.

Some children seek visual stimuli and enjoy watching flickering lights, shadow movements or bright colors. Allow the child to engage in meaningful visually stimulating activities, e.g. Where's Waldo?, Eye Spy or optical illusions books. Encourage them to use their visual interests to draw detailed maps, pictures, 3-D constructions or diagrams.

At times the visual stimuli can be so distracting for children that they lose the sequence of the activity in which they are involved. Use visual reminders such as cue cards or a sequence of pictures to help the child with the sequence of activities within the home, e.g. morning routine activities.

Children who are visually alert often want to talk about what they have seen immediately upon experiencing the event. They often are observing more things, and more rapidly than most children.

Encourage children to talk about what they have seen at a specific time rather than allowing constant interruption to respond to their observations. Help them to organize their visual impressions into a sequence before they talk by encouraging them to think about what is most important, what happened first, second, last.

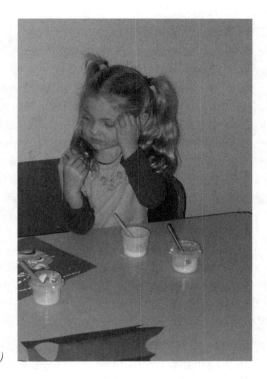

(a)

(b)

Figures 5.2a and b Bright or flashing lights and vivid colors may overwhelm some children who have visual sensitivities

Auditory sensitivities

Auditory senses are those senses responsive to sound. Some children are highly sensitive to the range of sounds (high, low, loud, echo) as well as the quantity (prolonged loud noise in a gymnasium or a mall). At times, the child may appear to manage in the situation, but later fall apart outside the noisy environment. Other children are unresponsive to sound – needing to be called a number of times, to be spoken to while directly facing them or needing to be specifically taught recognition of sounds that are used for safety purposes. An assessment by a speech and language pathologist for language and auditory processing difficulties may be necessary to help define causes of disorders of auditory responsiveness on either end of the continuum.

Questions to consider

1. What kinds of sounds are distressing for the child – loud, piercing, cumulative, competing, background noises such as buzzing fluorescent lights, fans, furnaces, refrigerators, or specific noises such as flushing of the toilet?

2. Does the child find certain music or singing enjoyable but other kinds distressing, e.g. upset by singing of the Happy Birthday song by children or adults singing off key?

3. Does the child enjoy noise and seek more or want to decrease or stop the noise?

4. Does the child react negatively to situations such as being in a gymnasium, indoor swimming pool, ball room in a children's play area of a restaurant, where there may be echo as well as excessive noise?

5. Does the child's overall state of arousal affect his tolerance to sound, e.g. can the child generally cope with sounds when calm but is more reactive when upset, excited, sick or tired?

6. Does the child complain about the loudness of others' voices but have a loud voice himself?

7. Does the child hear sounds, e.g. a siren, long before others can hear the sound?

8. Do instructions or information frequently have to be repeated for the child?

9. Does the child need to be faced directly while being spoken to?

10. Does the child ignore safety or directional sounds, e.g. classroom bells, road crossing signals for the blind, ambulance siren?

Management strategies

As much as possible try to predict and warn the child about noises that may occur, e.g. the noise in a shopping area or a garage, the school bell.

For sudden, unpredictable noises, teach children to use strategies such as covering their ears when an ambulance or fire truck goes by (see Figure 5.3). Develop self-talk phrases for sudden noises such as: "The fire truck is going to help the people."

Devise alternatives so noise-filled areas can be avoided if the child must accompany an adult to noisy places, e.g. the child could go to the library in the mall, go to the babysitting area in the mall or have one adult stay with the child and walk in the park while the other adult shops.

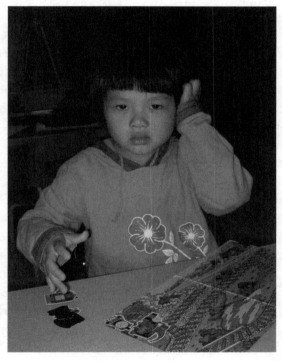

Figure 5.3 Sudden loud noises may be overwhelming for the child with auditory sensitivities

However, participating in activities in noisy environments is often unavoidable. In these situations lessening the sound by putting cotton or ear plugs in the child's ears (as long as this does not create a safety issue) is an option. Use headphones of calming music to block out irritating environmental sounds or have the child wear earmuffs in the winter when outside on a playground or in loud noisy activities such as tobogganing, skating or snowball fights where children are shrieking in fun.

Some noises such as a flushing toilet seem particularly irritating to children with RDSP. To manage this, have the child flush the toilet and walk immediately to the washroom door or go outside with another adult while the toilet is flushed. Don't insist on flushing for urination and hand washing can occur after the flush is through.

Another auditory irritant is often found at birthday parties. Tape record the Happy Birthday song so it can be played rather than having children singing off key.

Although children with an RDSP that involves auditory responses are often distressed by loud volume, screechy noises or prolonged sound, they frequently have little awareness of their own loud voices. Develop hand signs for adults to use to help direct the child's attention to listen, to lower their voice or to speak up. Make a video and/or tape of another child's voice in a social situation to help them understand loudness, softness, inside and outside voices. Turn up the volume on the TV or radio so they can hear really loud, outside voices, inside voices, and quiet voices. Practice voice volume when they are not around other adults or children. Talk about when it is a good time to yell – for example, stranger-danger, emergencies, if you are hurt.

Some children have low arousal to sounds and appear inattentive to auditory tasks and unresponsive to others in their environment. Helping these children to recognize that a large part of learning occurs through what we hear is important. Make a list of activities and decide what senses are used to complete each activity to help the child appreciate the role of senses in his life. Encourage alertness to sounds in nature and add auditory stimuli to common events, e.g. a tuneful bell to announce supper. Combine visual and auditory stimuli for learning tasks, such as singing the alphabet. Include fun listening tasks throughout the day, for example, recorded books, listening to a taped letter from Grandma, dancing to music, learning a children's song. Encourage the use of musical instruments, such as a toy xylophone, harmonica, bells, recorder, triangle, simple drumming. Discuss high and low sounds, loud and soft sounds.

Tactile sensitivities

Tactile sensations are received from touch initiated by oneself, others or objects. Some children are highly reactive to touch, while others are under-responsive and need alerting or visual clues to respond.

Questions to consider

1. Does the child dislike having his hair or nails cut?

2. Does the child complain about the texture of certain foods?

3. Does the child complain about the feel of certain textiles, or tags on clothing or seams in socks?

4. Does the child insist on wearing the same clothes every day or become upset until clothes are well washed and soft?

5. Is the child reactive to light touch such as the use of a comb for hair care or if someone rests a hand on the child's head?

6. Is the child reactive to children standing in a line behind or in front of him?

7. Does the child annoy others by touching them and getting into their space?

8. Does the child seek out tactile experiences by mouthing or touching objects as a way to learn about them?

Management strategies

Children who are negatively reactive to tactile stimulation often let their dislike be known in loud, long protests and physical avoidance. A number of predictive strategies can help avoid these reactions. Always ensure that the clothes purchased for the child can be returned if they are bought without the child present. However, the child may decide the clothes are fine in the store but, when they wear them and move about, find them irritating. Purchase clothing that is extra warm for the weight, such as fleece jackets or Gore-tex® raingear. Cut off tags from clothes and wear socks inside out, change from long-sleeved clothing to short sleeves or vice versa depending on the child's sensitivities. Investigate where to purchase seam-free underwear. The need to wear the same clothes can be accommodated by buying several outfits of the same style and material so they can be washed without the child having to wear other clothes that create sensory distress (see Figures 5.4a and b).

Adults touching the child need to learn to use firm pressure. Use a brush with firm rubber bristles and press firmly when brushing or washing their hair. Cut hair at night when the child is asleep, or allow longer than normal hair. Before the child begins activities that require touching various textures, the adult can apply deep pressure by placing their hands over the child's hands (or the child's hands between adult hands) and pressing down firmly.

Helping the child to learn language to explain his responses or to be predictive in situations to avoid being touched is important. Teach the child what to say, without anger, if they do not want to be touched. Practice saying the words before they need to use the script.

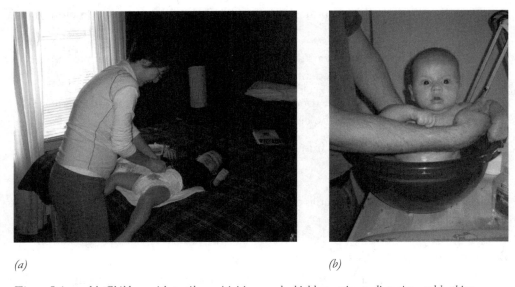

(a)   *(b)*

Figure 5.4a and b Children with tactile sensitivities may be highly reactive to diapering and bathing activities

Allow the child to apply his own suntan lotion or use heavier than usual pressure to apply it to the child. Encourage children to dry themselves with towels of varying texture in strong, vigorous movements.

Involve the child in theater, ballet, yoga or martial arts to become aware of his own body in space and learn responses to touching others or being touched. Provide the instructor with information related to the child's possible reactions and adaptations that may need to be made before and during class.

Some children with RDSP seek tactile stimulation even though they may dislike other children in their space or touching them. This becomes problematic when they invade others' personal space, kiss or touch others inappropriately. Teach the child about each person's "personal bubble" to help them judge personal distance. Place the child on a rotary balance board so the child can see that the world is all around him. Give visual boundaries by using a hula hoop to demonstrate the arm's length personal bubble.

The need to touch things can be encouraged in learning situations by pointing out that it is another sense through which we gain information. Provide opportunities to learn through touching objects of a wide variety of textures if the child seeks touch. Increase tactile opportunities for learning perceptual and motor skills such as drawing shapes on velvet or crawling on rough carpet.

Gustatory and olfactory sensitivities

Gustatory (taste) and olfactory (smell) sensory responses most often affect the eating behaviors of children with RDSP. Some children also have difficulty with oral motor control or engage in excessive chewing of clothing or objects or react strongly to smells within the environment.

Questions to consider

1. Does the child refuse to eat food that other children of the same age are eating?

2. Does the child gag, vomit or spit out food that has texture, spicy tastes, is either hot or cold?

3. Does the child seek out highly spiced food to eat or smell?

4. Does the child have a very limited diet (e.g. bland, soft foods, white foods, no meat, vegetables or fruit) or crave certain foods?

5. Does the child sniff food before eating or sniff objects as a way of exploring them?

6. Does the child react extremely to strong smells such as new paint, diapers, cleaning fluids, restaurant smells?

7. Does the child try to eat non-edible food – chewing on plastic, clothes, and sticks?

8. Does the child chew excessively on articles of clothing or objects?

9. Does the child drool excessively or breathe through the mouth or sit with his mouth open?

Please refer to Chapter 7, Physiological Responses, for suggestions related to management of food preferences and eating problems. Oral motor problems with swallowing, gagging and drooling should be addressed by assessment and treatment suggestions given by an occupational therapist or speech and language pathologist knowledgeable in oral motor remediation.

Management strategies

Try to be predictive of the environment, for example do not visit friends who have just painted their house, and do not walk through the perfume section in a store.

Introduce a variety of smells gradually and in an enticing way, e.g. the smell of cinnamon buns if your child will eat sticky buns. Make a game of introducing a variety of smells (see Figure 5.5). Put spices, fresh grass, seaweed, etc., in small opaque jars and have the child guess the smell, then have the child put in different-smelling objects and the parent guess what they are.

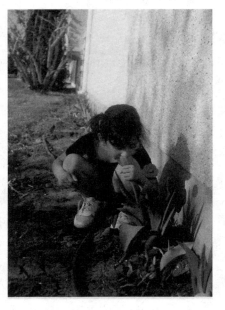

Figure 5.5 Children with olfactory sensitivities may be highly reactive to smells that occur in the environment

Allow children to hold their nose or pull a sweater over their nose when in high-smell situations. Provide a hanky with a smell on it that the child likes (e.g. a peppermint or chocolate smell) so the child can hold it to his nose when in unpleasant smelly environments.

For children who are not alert to smells or tastes play "guess the smell" games or a smelling version of I Spy (I smell) with different objects such as lemons, peppermint, fresh cut grass. Train the child to recognize dangerous smells, e.g. the smell of burning cloth or food, and to call an adult when the child smells these odors. Specifically teach the child with low smell arousal to recognize and eliminate smells that are unpleasant to others, e.g. dirty socks, farts, unbrushed teeth, rotting food.

A need to be constantly chewing or sucking on something is not only unhygienic, but also may lead to dental problems and, as the children get older, to teasing. To substitute for clothing, fingers or other objects provide chewable plastic tubing, some of which comes in animal or other shapes and as pencil toppers to make it more child friendly. To respond to the oral needs of a child who is constantly chewing, include food items for snacks and meals that require crunching (e.g. celery), chewing (e.g. beef jerky), blowing (e.g. use of straws in milkshake), and sucking (e.g. fruit popsicles).

Proprioceptive sensitivities

Proprioception is the sensory response to deep pressure, vibration, and muscle and joint movement. Some children seek out activities that provide them with deep pressure or joint movement. Such behaviors may make them appear unusual, e.g. flapping of hands (often at times of high anxiety) or deliberately running and bumping into objects with force.

If proprioceptive sensory information from muscles, joints and tendons is received and/or processed in a disorganized manner, the child may have immature motor responses and movements.

Questions to consider

1. Does the child seek out pressure by giving or asking for strong hugs, pushing into others or objects or jumping and thumping his feet?

2. Does the child enjoy activities such as jumping on a trampoline for long amounts of time?

3. Does the child frequently bump into objects or people as though on purpose?

4. Does the child bite on hard objects, himself or other people?

5. Does the child walk on tip toes, even when wearing shoes?

6. When playing or helping with activities, does the child seem to have less strength than other children the same age?

7. Does the child enjoy or fear appliances that vibrate such as the vacuum, hair drier, and blender?

Management strategies

With children who have RDSP, seeking or rejecting proprioceptive input can be observed in behaviors which may make them stand out among their peers or result in them being disciplined for intrusive behaviors.

Give the child something to hold in his hands that the child can press (stress ball or koosh ball or small smooth stone) to provide sensation and an opportunity to use pressure. For foam objects, ensure that the object is not easy to pick apart. Having something in the child's hands will also decrease ability to pick his nose if this is a sensory-seeking behavior.

Provide "heavy" work by encouraging the child to help push or move chairs and tables. When outside, encourage the child to run, jump over low objects, pull or push a wagon. Have the child move small rocks in the garden. Go for short steep hikes with the child.

Experiment with the use of weighted vests for periods of time when the child needs to attend. Vests should only be used for short periods of time with breaks in between use.

Encourage play activities such as animal walks (like a heavy elephant, like a hippopotamus), wheelbarrow walks, push-ups, tug of war with ropes, to allow for muscle and joint sensory input.

When sitting at a table or computer or when playing board games, have the child do push-ups in his seat by placing his hands at the side of the chair and push up or lean towards a wall and do wall push-ups.

Teach the child to ask for a hug rather than running up to others and squeezing them hard. Have the child experience a hard hug and a soft hug to help him differentiate. Use play dough to show what happens if something is squeezed too hard.

Vestibular sensitivities

Vestibular input from the inner ear directs protective, righting and equilibrium reactions. The vestibular system provides the basic reference point to space and gravity and the framework for the interpretation of the other sensations the brain receives (Ayers 1994). Some children have difficulty integrating vestibular input with other senses and so appear clumsy and uncoordinated or over- or under-sensitive to movement.

Questions to consider

1. Does the child have difficulty with balance activities?

2. Does the child appear clumsy and uncoordinated?

3. Does the child seek out, resist or reject activities that involve swinging or movement in space?

4. Does the child become carsick or dislike the movement of elevators?

5. Is the child afraid of heights and afraid of falling?

6. Does the child have difficulty with skipping or hopping?

For children who seek movement (see Figure 5.6):

1. Is the child a thrill seeker, wanting more and excessive movements such as swinging, twirling, and jumping?

2. Does the child find it hard to sit still – sitting on legs, wiggling or standing up and moving during meals and lessons?

3. Does the child enjoy swinging, slides and amusement rides for long periods of time?

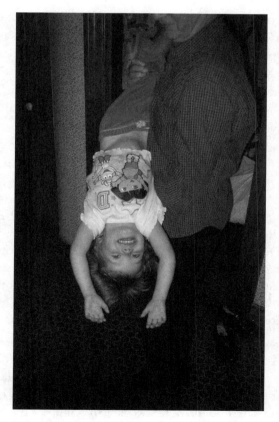

Figure 5.6 Some children with vestibular sensitivities seek prolonged and vigorous movement

Management strategies

Ensure that the child has adult help if he does not have adequate balance and grasp skills to maintain safe balance and movement when engaging in the suggested activities.

Encourage play on swings, monkey bars, climbing frames when the child is at school at recess or in free play family time. End the activity before the play period ends so the child can have time to prepare for the transition to return to class or home. Use somersaults, rolling and mat play as well as obstacle courses in gym work or on the carpet at home. Encourage the child to walk along low balance beam type of objects (curbs, low walls) as long as it is a safe height and environment. Hold his hand when learning this skill. Have the child walk in the spaces between the rungs of a ladder that is placed on the ground. Play games such as follow the leader with movement in all levels as part of the game. Teach the child to bounce and learn moves on a trampoline in supervised environments. Play catch and throw ball games with the child in a kneeling position. Play tug of war with ropes or ties.

Within the home, community or classroom, use a small exercise ball for the child to sit on to watch TV, listen to stories or during singing classes. Provide an inflatable Move 'n' Sit pillow for meals and class time. Allow the child to stand during homework or lessons, lie on his stomach when watching TV or change position for reading. Have the child stand at an easel when painting or drawing.

Consultation with a physiotherapist and/or an occupational therapist to develop a comprehensive movement program specific to the child's needs may be appropriate.

Summary

- In 2005, when revisions in the ZERO TO THREE diagnostic categories were finalized, the name Regulation Disorders of Sensory Processing was chosen to replace Regulation Disorders. This was in response to an increased awareness of a need to emphasize the impact of the various senses when processed by children with Regulation Disorders. Sensory inputs are often subtle or so fast that they are overlooked as a potential cause of reactive behaviors, avoidance, or inattention by children in academic, self-care and play situations.

- Management strategies require that caregivers analyze the preceding and present environment and activity, consider the sensory input that occurred and motor expectations and observe how the child reacted both before, during and after the event. Adaptations, modifications and remediation can then be planned to help the child to respond to sensory input or avoid aversive sensations.

Chapter 6

MOTOR RESPONSES

The development of motor responses

Most children develop their fine and gross motor skills in a predictable fashion. Babies learn to bring their hands together to be able to play and hold their bottle or cup. Development of the ability to point and use a pincer grip gives infants independence in indicating specific objects and learning more about them. Crawling and then walking allows exploration of their environment. Each motor skill requires coordination of both large and fine motor muscles, as well as processing visual, vestibular, kinesthetic and proprioceptive input. In addition, an adequate awareness of the spatial relations of one's own body parts and a motor memory for movements adds to the development of competence in activities requiring motor responses.

By diagnostic definition, children who have Regulation Disorders of Sensory Processing (RDSP) also have motor problems. Sometimes the term "dyspraxic" is applied to their responses. This means they have difficulty planning and performing activities requiring motor responses. These problems may be apparent in awkwardness in the skills of everyday life, e.g. tying shoelaces, using a fork and spoon, dressing, or clumsiness in tasks requiring balance, or in movement and/or balance when running, climbing or using athletic equipment. These types of motor problems are not unique to children with RDSP. Children with learning disabilities, Attention Deficit Hyperactivity Disorder (ADHD) and autism are also frequently noted to have coordination problems along with other symptoms related to their primary condition. Other neurological problems such as mild cerebral palsy may result in motor problems that appear similar to the altered motor responses of children without this condition. A specific diagnosis of Developmental Coordination Disorder indicates that a child has a primary disability that substantially affects their daily functioning, related to either or both fine and gross motor coordination.

Questions to consider

1. In general, can the child complete fine and gross motor tasks at a level similar to her peers?

2. Does the child avoid or have difficulty with gross motor activities involving balance, speed or coordination?

3. Does the child avoid or have difficulty with fine motor activities involving small objects that require a pincer (three-point) grip or (age three or older) involving use of crayons, pencils, paint brushes, finger games such as Itsy Bitsy Spider?

4. Does the child have difficulty with age-appropriate self-help tasks such as dressing, feeding herself or bathing and bathroom skills?

5. Can the child complete a sequence of motor activities, e.g. remember the movements necessary to turn book pages, open a container, bat a ball?

6. Does the child know the names of her body parts and their spatial relationship to one another, e.g. my ears are at the side of my head?

7. Does the child know to name and to respond to spatial words such as under, over, in, on, between, in front of, beside, behind?

8. Does the child prefer large or repetitive motor movements to small refined movements?

9. Does the child have excessive interest in or seek out activities such as spinning, rocking, or repetitive movements?

10. Is the child afraid of being swung up in the air or having her feet off the ground?

11. Does the child have difficulty adjusting to changes in position and appear to use vision to compensate for positional change?

12. Does the child appear slow, clumsy or awkward when moving or completing tasks?

13. Does the child require constant supervision to be physically safe?

Management strategies – gross motor skills

Children with motor problems can improve in their skill levels (see Figures 6.1a and b). The child's motivation to learn a task goes a long way to helping her have the persistence to practice the activity enough to learn the component parts, the sequence and the reintegration of motor movements or to learn an alternate way to succeed.

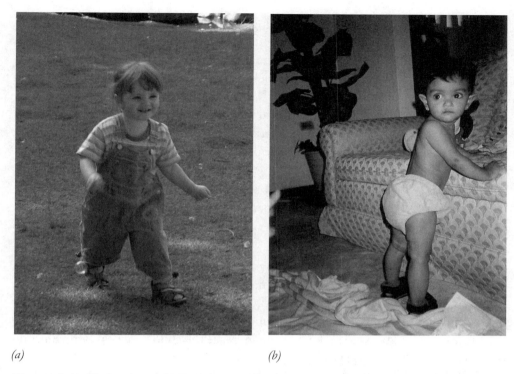

(a)   (b)

Figure 6.1a and b Gross motor skills may present problems for the child with Regulation Disorders

The first step is to identify if the task that the child is expected to complete is at an age-appropriate level. Does the child want to learn this task/activity or is it an adult's priority? Obviously an activity such as being able to feed oneself is important socially and in terms of independence, and allows better time management for all family members so is a high priority for parents. While learning to ride a bike may be a top priority as identified by the child, playing on a T-ball team may not be important.

Identifying the component parts of the activity and where the breakdown occurs in the child's performance will be necessary. Research at the CanChild Center for Childhood Disability Research, McMaster University, has demonstrated that by using a "top-down" cognitive model to approach motor learning tasks, children can learn activities that are difficult for them and generalize their learning. It is important for the children to choose the skills they want to learn and improve.

Using the cognitive model, the researchers taught children verbal self-guidance strategies to accomplish the goal they first defined, then developed a method to accomplish the plan, completed the plan and then checked the results (goal, plan, do, check). As well, adults used non-intrusive scaffolding to help the child accomplish the defined goal by guiding the child to discover alternatives if problems develop along the way. Children are encouraged to think, "Now I need a different plan" rather than that they are unable to do the task, when they meet a difficulty. See the website of CanChild in the Resources section for more information on this approach.

Consultation with a pediatric physical therapist for an assessment of the child's overall strength, flexibility, range of motion and balance often is useful. As well a pediatric physiotherapist can give advice on exercises to increase the child's endurance, balance and flexibility.

Management strategies – group sports

During the primary years, play in group sports is seldom a problem. The younger children are accepting of each other's differences and generally do not isolate children with poor skills. However, by intermediate grades (age nine to ten), children (and their parents) have become more competitive in sports, and more aware of, and often less tolerant of, individual differences. This may lead to the child with lingering aspects of RDSP being teased or left out of team sports. There are some considerations to make that can increase the child's success before a child is placed in an organized sport.

Talk to the child's coach or sensei if considering a team activity or martial arts. Have the child meet the leader and watch other children doing the activity before the child is committed to attending. Explain to the instructor the child's learning style, what causes extreme responses and what helps to calm her down. Ask if a parent can be present for the first few minutes of the classes at the beginning, to help the child transition into the new activity. Select sports that do not require complex movements if the child has motor coordination problems.

Consider the competitive level of the sport. In early years "team" sports may be successful with an understanding coach and accepting team mates. As the skill level requirements and the desire to win increases, monitor the responses of the child. Although a caring coach can make the difference in success for any child, there are also a variety of non-competitive sports that provide exercise and enjoyment for children and families.

With sports that require protective equipment such as teeth guards, or goggles, encourage the child to wear the equipment from the beginning to help develop skill (e.g. putting head under water/blowing bubbles) or tolerance of the feeling of something in one's mouth or over the face. Try out the equipment before the first day of practice so the child is aware of the feeling or restrictions. Create/define a safe place in the sporting situations or the gym where the child can go if activities become over-stimulating for her.

Non-competitive sports (or ones where you can compete against your own score) are often good choices for children with gross and fine motor challenges.

The following activities are non-competitive or can be used to increase time, score, and skills against one's own ability: swimming, bowling, catch and throw ball games, Velcro ball, riding a bike or scooter, distance walking, hiking, camping/backpacking, exercise programs designed for kids, yoga for children, snowshoeing, cross- country skiing, downhill skiing, Frisbee, Frisbee golf, playground equipment, horseback riding, orienteering, tobogganing, canoeing, kayaking, sailing. Some children respond well to the structure and repetition in martial arts programs.

Management strategies – fine motor skills

Motor movement problems may also affect a child's involvement in activities that require fine motor skills. This becomes most apparent when children are expected to draw, color, paint and write with pencils, crayons and paint brushes, and with self-care skills (see Figures 6.2a and b). It is useful to have a complete occupational therapy assessment of fine motor, perceptual and self-care skills, to define abilities and difficulties in these areas. The occupational therapist may recommend treatment and home exercises to help children develop age-appropriate muscle strength and discrimination in their arms, hands and finger muscles and to strengthen their shoulder muscles and trunk stability, since strength and dexterity in all of these areas helps with more refined hand and finger use.

Some considerations when expecting a child to complete fine motor/perceptual activities at home, school or in the community are:

- What perceptual and motor skills are required for the task(s)? Does the child have any problems in these areas?

- Is this activity at an appropriate age and interest level for the child?

- Is the child motivated to do this activity?

- How long does the activity take to complete? (Some children's performance deteriorates dependent on how long they are required to do the task, e.g. writing activities.)

Teachers or community leaders may need help to think of modifications or adaptations of equipment or the task to help the child to succeed. Analyze the task for perceptual and motor requirements and consider where any breakdown may occur. Use the "goal, plan, do, check" approach for completing tasks that are difficult because of fine motor/perceptual difficulties.

Within school settings, there are numerous technological aids that are available to help a child to complete writing and fine motor tasks. The most obvious one is use of a computer, but once again collaboration will need to occur with the school

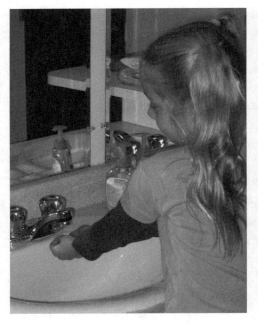
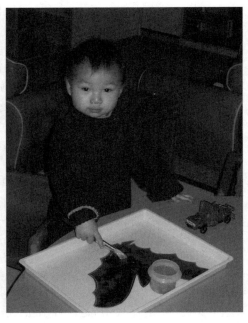

(a)   (b)

Figure 6.2a and b Fine motor problems may be seen in completion of self-care skills, and use of pencils and crayons

resource team to find what the school will provide, what support or instruction is available, and what is the best type of resource for the child's specific needs. Other less technical materials are adapted equipment such as pencil grips and specialized scissors.

Adapting and modifying the learning environment may be one of the biggest challenges. Ensuring that the child's motor needs are identified on the Individual Education Plan (IEP) is important so that teachers (or community instructors who you will need to inform) work together with parents to problem-solve the different approaches that may be needed so the child can have success in the same activities that her peers complete.

At home, use of track suits, Velcro closure on runners, lightweight tube socks (turned inside out if sensory issues exist) and large zipper closures are helpful for dressing skills. Large rubber grip spoon, knife and fork handles are helpful in the early years, and non-slip material under plates helps with stability when cutting food. An occupational therapist is a useful consultant for discussing adaptations that will help increase the child's independence if fine motor problems are severe and persistent.

Summary

- Both fine and gross motor responses develop in a fairly predictable sequence and are essential for self-care, academic and leisure activities. By definition, children with Regulation Disorders of Sensory Processing have some motor impairments.

- Recent research has demonstrated that using a "top-down" cognitive approach of "goal, plan, do, check" can help children to learn to improve selected motor skills. As well, adults will need to analyze motor tasks for sensory and perceptual requirements and help to develop adaptations and modifications that allow the child to participate with her peers in community, home and school activities that require motor skills.

Chapter 7

PHYSIOLOGICAL RESPONSES

The main physiological areas that result in problems for infants and young toddlers with Regulation Disorders of Sensory Processing (RDSP) are in the areas of eating, sleeping, elimination and the ability to self-calm. Maladaptive physiological responses may extend into preschool years with the children having such problems as sleeping difficulties, excessive sweating and restricted eating patterns.

To address these issues, because the baby cannot yet talk, the most important skill parents will need to develop is to learn to read the baby's body, verbalizations and movement cues.

There are also a number of shifts that can be made in the baby's environment or handling of them that may help them to self-calm or progress in the developmental tasks of eating, sleeping and elimination.

Management strategies to develop self-calming

A caregiver may try many ways to soothe a fretful baby. Approaches that parents of infants with RDSP have found helpful are to firmly wrap the very young baby (swaddling) while holding him and hold the baby firmly against the adult chest. Try moving the baby up and down to soothe – some babies respond to a vertical motion better than a rocking or side-to-side motion.

When on walks, use a "kangaroo carrier" or "Snuggly" that allows skin-to-skin contact for fretful babies (Feldman *et al.* 2002). Do not take the baby to stimulating environments such as malls or heavy traffic areas.

Sometimes taking the baby for a drive helps the baby to calm. Often the low frequency vibration motion of the car will soothe him. However, *never* leave your baby unattended and asleep in a car seat, in a child swing seat or on a dryer to jiggle them to sleep. Leaving a baby unattended and sleeping in a car seat has resulted in the death of several babies due to being caught in the straps.

Be alert to progression from laughter to hysteria as the baby gets wound up and is unable to calm. Help the child to calm by removing him from the stimulation, talking calmly, dimming the lights. Play soft instrumental or classical music when the baby is upset. Tapes of intrauterine sounds may help fussy babies who are not sleeping or who have a sleep/wake cycle reversed.

Give the baby a massage with a firm pressure. Some community centers have baby massage classes or a massage practitioner may teach you the skills.

Management strategies to develop sleep routines

Different families and cultures have expectations about when and how a baby should sleep. Co-sleeping (babies and parents) has been a controversial issue and certain sleeping patterns, including early independence in sleeping habits, are culture specific (McKenna *et al.* 1993). In addition, psychosocial factors such as the available sleeping places for the family members may dictate the sleeping patterns of infants.

Sleep literature about infant sleep is vast. We have provided some guidelines that may be particularly important for children with RDSP but many websites provide additional extensive information (Feldman *et al.* 2002; Ghaem *et al.* 1998; McKenna *et al.* 1993).

Organizing the baby's/child's room to provide a non-stimulating environment is important. Put the nursery in a back room where it is facing a quiet yard or less traffic. Use heavy curtains to keep out daylight for daytime naps. Remove pictures on walls and decals on cribs that may be visually irritating/stimulating to the baby. Shift the position of night lights until a positive effect is found. For older children, keep the room orderly by the use of cupboards and boxes with lids for storage of toys etc. to decrease distractions.

Encouraging regular patterns of sleep is important to help the child develop a predictable rhythm and pattern to his day and night time. Ensure that the infant or young child has had opportunity to move, play and be alert throughout the day so they do not need to extend activity into the night time. Arrange a quiet transition time between play and sleep times.

Some infants only need a short nap – others a longer time. Keep a record of the baby's sleep habits to see if there is a pattern emerging. Develop a routine for nap and sleep times – a similar time, place and involving relaxing activities such as a warm bath, a song, the same story every night. Have pictures of the sleep routine – bath, supper, play, story, sleeping in their own bed. Review these pictures with the child before beginning the routine. Photographs of the child doing each of the activities help the child to transfer the picture activity to real-life behaviors. Even with a baby, give him a warning that it will soon be sleep time and rehearse the routine. Encourage the child to sleep in his own bed rather than expecting to go to bed with adults and be transferred to their bed. If night-time crying occurs, calm the child in his own bed without taking him out of his bed. Gradually increase the time that you wait before going in to comfort the child and then stay only long enough to settle the child.

Do not use feeding in the middle of the night to calm the child – this can lead to disruption of daytime eating habits as well as tooth decay. Instead find a soft toy or "blanky" that is comforting for the child.

Changes and transitions are difficult times for children with RDSP – especially when they are tired or irritable before sleep time. If it is necessary to have the baby sleep in different environments, or beds (e.g. sleep in a portable crib for traveling), introduce the baby to the bed before sleep time and before you are traveling. When changing linen or covers, introduce them to the child during non-sleep times, e.g. use them on the floor during playtime to introduce the color, texture etc. before the child is expected to be calm when surrounded by them. Use soft background music or the white noise of a vacuum cleaner, or a hairdryer as a transition sound while the baby is going to sleep.

Tactile sensory reactions to the feel of pajamas and bedding may cause distress in some children. Try different materials such as stretch jersey or high thread count cotton which provides a smooth surface for bedding. Sleepers with or without feet, short or long pajamas or a nightdress of stretch materials or cotton etc. need to be explored. A visit to the local children's consignment store may provide a variety of nightwear without excessive cost. Some children are very warm all the time and do not need to wear very many night clothes.

Management strategies to regulate elimination patterns

Several websites give good basic strategies and recommended books for help with toilet training (see the Resources section). The suggestions included here are to address problems that have been described by parents as specific to children with RDSP.

Toilet training a child with RDSP may lead to the same struggles as occur in other aspects of the child's life that are dominated by sensory and affective issues. The baby and toddler may have low awareness of wetness versus dryness or may have lowered muscle tone resulting in difficulty in waiting to eliminate until they are in the toileting situation. From the earliest of ages the baby may be sensitive to the process of elimination and diapering.

Since dressing and undressing accompanies diapering or toileting, suggestions related to these issues in babies are included here. Diapering a wriggling baby can be frustrating at the best of times. Add a child who is sensitive to touch, feel of fabrics, smell or being put in various positions and it becomes a frequent challenge. Some suggestions to address this are to warm up diapers with a hairdryer or in the clothes dryer before putting them on the baby. Experiment with use of cloth diapers (softer and more pliable) rather than commercial disposable diapers.

Use non-perfumed baby wipes, and laundry soap or softeners without perfume. Use warm water on a washcloth and then the use of a towel for clean-ups, if the child does not like toilet paper for wiping, often helps. Using firm pressure when wiping or drying lessens reaction to light touch.

If the child is resistant to lying down to have diapers replaced, have him sit on them for closure, or put them on while standing.

Toilet training creates another challenge for both the parents and a child with RDSP. Balance, tactile, olfactory and auditory reactions may interfere with the process. When toilet training using a potty begins, there are several suggestions that may help increase the child's willingness to participate.

- Develop a toileting routine by tracking the child's bowel movements to see if there is a time pattern that can be followed when having him sit on the toilet. Have the child sit on the toilet immediately after eating and before going out of the house.

- Eliminate some of the tactile responses by use of a seat cover that is soft if placing a kiddy cover over an adult seat. Warm the seat cover with hot water and dry if the cold plastic bothers the child.

- Assess whether the child has adequate balance to sit on the adult seat with a cover or if a small child seat and potty will be more secure. Put a stool under the child's feet for an additional feeling of stability.

- Reinforce what the child is doing and why by reading a children's book related to toileting if the child is sitting for several minutes on the toilet.

- Have the child look when they are urinating so they experience the feeling and the action and see the result. If the flushing noise upsets the child, flush after they have left the room.

Dressing a baby and toddler presents many of the same sensory problems as diapering. To respond to tactile sensations put the clothing in the dryer to warm them before putting them on or, if the child is always warm, experiment to see if it is more acceptable to the child if the clothes are cool before they are put on. Use soft clothing or well-washed clothing rather than stiff baby jeans or materials.

Experiment to see if the baby responds better to close-fitting clothes and sleepers or looser clothing.

Management strategies for eating and mealtimes

The food intake of children is a highly emotional topic for most parents and family members. Feeding a baby or child is one of the most basic caregiving events. However, children with RDSP may begin life with difficulty nursing and resist the introduction of textured food. Some children insist on eating the same taste, texture and color of food.

A child's eating habits often are attributed to poor parenting. Other adults will readily provide their own favorite solution to "make" the child eat. As well, adults will frequently remark about the child's intake in front of the child at the table. These "helpful" suggestions are not helpful either to the child or the parents. To encourage the child to participate in and enjoy mealtimes and extend his food preferences, eating should be seen as an ordinary event that everyone does. Do not make an issue or give praise about what or how much food is eaten.

Encourage all family members to have a consistent approach and expectation in whatever living or caregiving situation they have (e.g. if parents are separated and living in two different homes or grandparents or daycare do part of the childcare). Write down what the eating routine is and the responses that are expected. Ensure that the child is moderately hungry when he is offered a meal.

Have specific mealtimes and snack times – do not have food or drink sitting out for grazing. Give milk and liquids at the meal or snack times so they do not fill up the child between meals. Use water for liquids between meals and snacks. Determine a specific amount of time for each meal or snack time. Do not force feed the child or leave the child sitting at the table for excessive amounts of time.

Make the mealtime an enjoyable time for everyone. Have family discussions and encourage the child to join in conversations. Do not make mealtime a playtime with toys and activities (except at a restaurant where the child has to wait for the meal).

Encourage independence in eating skills and this will also increase attention on the process (see Figures 7.1a and b). Anticipate new situations that may disrupt established eating routines. If the child is going to be eating in a new situation or there are visitors to the home, where the adults do not know about the child's eating preferences, brief them ahead of time and ask them to not comment at all on the food or the child's eating. If necessary, take a prepared meal that can be heated up for the child's meal when visiting or at a restaurant.

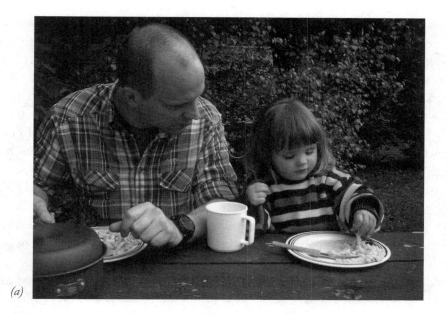

(a)

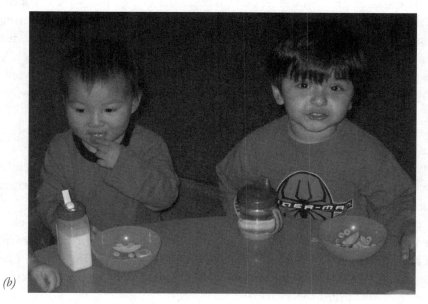

(b)

Figure 7.1a and b Provision of easy finger foods and child-sized dishes encourages feeding oneself

If the child has extremely limited food preferences, consultation with a nutritionist is advised. Ask the family doctor for a referral to a public health unit dietician or to a dietician at the local children's hospital. Inform relatives (especially grandparents) that consultation with a dietician or doctor has occurred and everyone is ensuring that the child has adequate and appropriate intake.

Use blended foods such as putting soya milk for protein in a milk shake. Add blended vegetables to tomato sauce, meatloaf, hamburgers.

Introduce new foods very gradually and in very small amounts. Use food that is a similar texture and color to foods that are tolerated. Encourage a one-taste test for new tastes rather than expecting the child to eat a lot of any new food item.

Preschool and school-age children enjoy helping prepare meals. This may motivate them to eat the food they have helped to prepare.

If the child appears unaware of taste differences, include alerting food items such as fruit popsicles that are sour, spicy foods such as flavored rice crackers, and dipping sauces. For treats, use unique objects that have different tastes, e.g. turquoise candy canes, multishaped rice crackers, nuts and bolts party mix to encourage exploring tastes.

Children with RDSP often limit the taste, color and texture of foods that they eat. Do not make eating a variety of food into a daily battlefield. Over time the majority of children gradually shift and increase their tolerance to new foods.

If the child has a predominant gag reflex when eating (gags or vomits during or after eating), will only eat soft-textured food or drools excessively, assessment and management recommendations by an occupational therapist or speech and language therapist trained in feeding problems will be of use. Useful books related to helping solve food preferences and eating problems are listed in the Resources section.

Olfactory (smell) responses may also affect the child's interest in eating or he may react to being in settings that have high smells or scents. If the child has a high sensitivity to smells, tastes, textures and chewing needs, encourage the child to smell, feel and taste the new food for several meals before eating it. Serve generally bland-smelling food.

Oral motor needs are often shown by the child constantly chewing on clothes or fingers. They may find the oral motor activity calming or have a need for strong motor activity and deep oral pressure obtained from strong chewing. Sturdy plastic tubes specifically designed for high-impact chewing are available from specialized companies (see resources section).

Summary

- The dysregulated physiological responses of a baby, toddler or child with Regulation Disorders of Sensory Processing can cause as much distress for their parents as for themselves. Embedded in both tradition and cultural values, the focus on sleeping, eating and elimination patterns has a family history and emotion component unlike any of the other problems presented by these children. In planning interventions, it is essential to consider the family context as well as analyzing the environment and sensory and motor influences. Management strategies that utilize adaptations and modifications are useful. Routines help lessen anxiety for the child, and encourage the adults in the child's life to not make a fuss about the events, resulting in everyone being able to self-calm.

Chapter 8

BEHAVIORAL ORGANIZATION AND PROCESSING – AFFECT REGULATION

Brain development in affect regulation and processing

Affect regulation means regulating your mood and feelings. The word *affect* is usually used to denote any emotional state, both pleasant and unpleasant, and suggests a general mood state (Laplanche and Pontalis 1973). Children with Regulation Disorders of Sensory Processing (RDSP) often have enormous difficulties with regulating their emotions so discussion about this domain is important.

Emotional regulation and processing is mediated by the autonomic nervous system (the system in our brain over which we have limited control and that initiates such responses as sneezing, coughing, and sweating) which consists of sympathetic and parasympathetic pathways. Both sympathetic and parasympathetic nerve pathways play a part in self-regulation. Response by sympathetic pathways leads to activity such as increased heart rate and respiration, and to energy-consuming activity. Parasympathetic activity leads to a decrease in heart rate and respiration, numbness, and shutting down, with energy conservation and decreased thinking activity.

Simultaneous activation of parasympathetic and sympathetic pathways may lead to emotions such as explosive rage. Higher functions are shut down, rational thought becomes impossible and a more primitive, reflexive mode of response (driven by the limbic system, our most primitive response system) replaces the higher levels of responding.

The human brain has evolved with specialized capacities originating in or responding to the different functions of the frontal, parietal, temporal and occipital brain lobes. The frontal lobes are concerned with reasoning, problem-solving, planning, emotions, speech and movement.

The frontal lobes of the brain are connected with the limbic system so the emotional regulation of arousal and expression of emotions starts very early in life. There is a rapid brain growth in the postnatal period and it is mostly experience dependent. The experiences (e.g. mother–infant relational experiences) allow growth and grouping of the neurons in the brain. The experiences have another important function, which is "pruning" or discarding of unused connections (Schore 2003). Thus regulatory processes are not always proceeding in one direction. These processes of growth of neurons, and discarding of unused connections, are important for the development of brain functions called executive functions. Executive functions help detect meaning from one's environment by developing the ability to define a problem, devise a plan to solve the problem and evaluate the result of carrying out the plan.

Self-regulation of behavior, including management of emotions, begins before speech develops, with the ability to regulate and inhibit behavior generally being accomplished by age three. Self-regulation of cognitive processes needed for problem-solving, attention control, intentionality, development of private speech and anticipation (skills which are needed for behavioral control) is achieved as the prefrontal cortex area of the brain matures. From the age of five years, there is usually a noticeable increase in self-regulation and therefore an anticipated increase in emotional and behavioral control (Calkins 2000; Calkins and Howse 2004; Porges *et al.* 1996; Schore 2003; Siegel 1999).

Emotional regulation is an important developmental milestone that needs to be mastered to become a well-functioning individual. In children with RDSP, the high intensity of emotions or the low arousal of the minimally involved child both signify difficulties in attaining this developmental milestone.

Dimensions of emotional regulation

When observing the emotional responses of children with RDSP, children who over-react or under-react to a situation are often seen.

Some children seek out high-stimulation activities and events (see Figures 8.1a and b). Children with the opposite tendency do not seem to be aware of the situation and possible responses to it. These children often also have difficulty in interpretation of, and responding to, the emotions of others – either misinterpreting the emotion, perseverating on the experience or ignoring others' expression of emotion.

Analysis of the child's behaviors can lead to intervention that will help her to respond more appropriately. To do this, it is useful to know the dimensions or facets that contribute to emotional regulation.

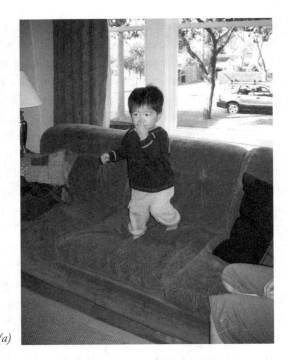

(a)

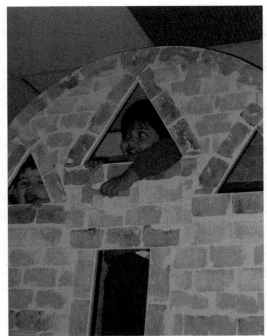

(b)

*Figures 8.1a and b Some children with Regulation
Disorders seek out high-stimulation activities or events*

Emotions can be both *regulating* – they help us to respond emotionally to others and our environment (e.g. a child is sad because he has received a time-out) – and *regulated* – the emotions are changed by the individual (e.g. a baby or toddler reduces stress by sucking on its thumb for self-soothing) (Cole, Martin and Dennis 2004).

Sroufe refers to the development and expression of affect and then management of the emotions that developed as the "twin tasks" of emotion (Sroufe 1999, p. 156).

Siegel (1999) simplifies the brain connections required to do the twin tasks of regulating and regulated emotions. He describes a combination of factors that includes *intensity* that is linked with the arousal and appraisal system. For example, imagine a child Peter, with RDSP, who saw a funny movie, and started to laugh. However, his enjoyment lasts long after the other children's and now he is rolling on the floor with tears in his eyes, all in a pleasant mood state. As he continues, he may get so worked up that he pushes his little sibling and now a cycle of unnecessary conflict is initiated. This same child may have difficulty controlling his angry feelings and reactions and so the conflict escalates.

Another child, Travis, hears the ice-cream truck playing his favorite song. He waits excitedly and happily on the front lawn of his house with his older sister, with money in his hand that he got for his birthday. Today, the ice-cream truck does not stop. It is nobody's fault, but Travis is inconsolable. He sobs so hard and thrashes around so violently that the neighbors gather around him, looking at his sister suspiciously, in case she was harsh with him. When Travis recognizes there is a crowd, his behavior becomes even more aroused and he screams even louder.

For each of these children, the intensity of both happy and angry feelings rapidly escalated to an out-of-control state. It is this intensity of emotions that set them apart from other children who may also be situationally affected.

A second dimension of emotional regulation that Siegel describes is the *threshold of response* in the active management of emotions. This threshold is influenced by the experiences each person has, the neurological responses children are born with (e.g. the sensitive child) and the responses children learn from parents who may transmit their own sensitivities and fears to their children.

Siegel also introduces the dimension of *windows of tolerance* that is central to our understanding of why children with RDSP are not able to modulate their emotions. These "windows of tolerance" are the amount and degrees of emotion that each person can handle. If the emotional arousal moves beyond the boundaries of what a child can tolerate, then the child is clearly in need of help from others in managing these emotions (Siegel 1999, pp. 246–58).

It is important to note parents' descriptions of their child acting like a "Jekyll and Hyde" if she does not get enough sleep or food. They may have some credence, as we are learning through vagal stimulation research (Porges *et al.* 1996). Hunger and exhaustion can both alter these "windows of tolerance."

Some children with RDSP avoid moderate to high emotional responses and withdraw or appear unresponsive. These children need help in experiencing emotional responses that have both variety and intensity.

The development of emotional regulation

The development of emotional self-regulation usually occurs in a predictable fashion. In the newborn, social, emotional and cognitive development go hand in hand. The baby learns to smile in response to a smiling or familiar face, laugh when tickled, and cry when hungry or afraid.

During the first year the caregiver role is important. It is by the circles of communication (e.g. the baby coos, the caregiver imitates the sound and smiles at the baby, the baby smiles and coos again) that the child learns the interactive nature of emotional responses (see Figure 8.2). As well, it is by the development of attachment to a caregiver, and the loving responses extended by the caregiver, that the early origins of the ability to emotionally care for self and others is developed.

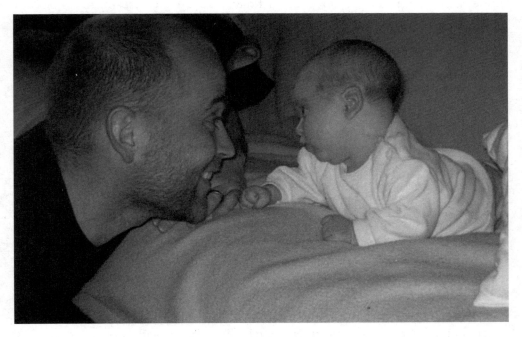

Figure 8.2 A father and son complete circles of communication

During the second year, as a toddler, the child develops symbolic thought and voluntary control over at least some of their emotions. Play with toys begins to include some fantasy and representation of the emotions and behaviors that the child sees within their daily life. Firm and responsive parenting is important as the child begins to test exactly what results a temper tantrum can give, or judge the adult responses to out-of-control laughter.

Preschoolers and kindergarten children begin to have true internal self-regulation of behaviors and emotions. They can internalize rules and develop strategies and plans when playing and responding to peers and adults. Although they need less constant adult supervision, the adults in their lives need to provide context for the child by pointing out what others are doing, encouraging perspective-taking and help to interpret social and emotional language. By providing these bridges, the adult helps to facilitate problem-solving and the child's efforts at self-regulation.

Many of the children with RDSP do not seem to get joy from living or from their environment, in the way one hopes children will enjoy life. Parents are distressed to see their child assume such an angry or sad stance about life.

Children with RDSP do show well-timed emotionality but may demonstrate it with greater intensity and duration than other children. They are able to show empathy but may become stuck on the feeling or event and ask or comment over and over about what they saw or experienced. When children are physically ill they may want more of everything – attention, food, and assurances of safety.

Parents have concern that their children may become victimized because of their difficulty in managing their own behavior, expressing their feelings and problem-solving. These are valid concerns since their children's unusual style of responsiveness make them stand apart from their peers. Education of peers, educators and the children themselves to help develop social skills and social problem-solving is essential.

Children with RDSP often have very intense reactions to events, feelings or sensory input. They get really excited, have extreme laughter, or become very physical in activity. This is part temperament, part genetic, and part experience dependent, which interacts with the children's unique responses to sensory input. As time goes by, usually their intense responses modify. Often when they are young they need help in putting the brakes on their own feeling responses – either happiness or anger. When the children are young and show extreme positive emotional responses, most people do not mind, but as they get older if they demonstrate anger with the same intensity, then people become worried.

Some children kiss very hard, scratch in happiness, hug with excessive strength and may appear aggressive in their interactions. They may have extremes of pain thresholds – either responding in the extreme themselves to minor injuries or not appearing to feel pain at all. Parents have also observed their children make rapid switches in intensity of play. Children's behavior may be in response to sound or other sensory overload or because they have a sensory need. Children's laughter in these situations may be because they do not know how to react and are anxious.

They will be highly interested in a topic and then suddenly switch to disinterest. This difficulty with behavioral and emotional regulation also makes it difficult for the parents to react appropriately since at times the behaviors rapidly escalate to defiance. It is important that parents think about behavioral management strategies before their children's tantrums and out-of-control behavior occur.

Attachment and self-regulation

Ideally, secure attachment to one's primary caregiver(s) paves the path for adequate social and emotional adjustment in life, assuming other factors, such as physical health and psychosocial events, are optimal. The social context and experiences within their family increases children's feelings of safety and security and therefore allows them to organize their emotions more effectively.

Having secure attachment in infancy and early childhood alone does not guarantee positive emotional health throughout life. We do know, however, that having insecure or disorganized attachment experiences will affect a child's socio-emotional adjustment. If the child has experienced terror early in life, the sensation of being out of control without having someone to help organize her emotions may create long-term distress (Main and Hesse 1990).

Emotional engagement and attachment enhances learning, while disengagement inhibits learning. In the past, attachment was construed as either secure or insecure attachment. Now, another category defined as Disorganized Attachment (Main and Hesse 1990) is reserved for children who are unable to follow a particular style of relating, with responses that are either contradictory or repetitive and often exhibiting aggressive behavior.

In Disorganized Attachment the core problem in the mother–child relationship that may affect the child's attachment is that the caregiver is perceived as frightened or frightening to the infant (a mother who herself is abused and distressed, or an angry, aggressive mother). This gives rise to contradictory behaviors in the infant such as freezing or aggression without provocation. If this caregiver behavior occurs, it needs to be one of the factors that is considered and incorporated in the management of the child with RDSP. Indeed, this development of a protective shield for the child, originating from the development of secure attachment between caregiver and child, and having a "good fit" between parent and child, is the foundation of most therapies for children who have attachment difficulties (Erickson 1999; Juffer, Bakermans-Kranenburg and Van Ijzendoom 2005; Karen 1994; Lyons-Ruth, Alpern and Repacholi 1993; Porges *et al.* 1996).

Parental modeling of emotional regulation, and support for emotional recovery, is very important. For instance, if adults are speaking in an angry voice, the child's voice will often get louder and more high-pitched too. If parents react with erratic emotional responses, the child may not learn appropriate responses to events. The parents may need to help the child regulate herself in situations of intense emotions (e.g. if the child has a tantrum, the parents need to model self-calming methods). Children with RDSP need a supportive, reflective, guiding person to help with emotional regulation.

Management strategies for aggressive/happy/tantrum behaviors

Children with RDSP often have more intense responses (both positive and negative) to events or other people than their peers (see Figures 8.3a and b).

While these responses may be tolerated in babies and toddlers – often interpreted as "just a stage" – when they continue into preschool age and early school-age children, the behaviors bring negative responses to both the child and the parents.

Every child needs help in developing the ability to be aware of the feelings of others – the origins of empathy. To encourage development of this skill, take pictures of the child and family members in different situations and showing different feelings – sad, mad, happy, scared, excited – so these faces provide familiar cues for the child. Talk about the possible context of these feelings and comment when others are seen demonstrating the feeling. Use a "How are you feeling today?" chart that family members can change to match their feelings. Ask and comment about the feelings of characters in books, videos and movies.

Children need help and support in learning to take the perspective of other children. This is an age-related developmental skill. At age five and six a child is just beginning to develop thinking about the feelings of others at a more complex level. Although children may feel remorse about some interaction they may be so stressed by the incident that they don't want to talk about it. An expression of "sorry" may be said quickly but with little meaning. If the child cannot describe another child's possible feelings, give her the probable answer and describe what made you think that (facial expression, tone of voice, body language, etc.).

When the child has what appears to be an impulsive display of anger or aggression, analyze the problem behavior(s) that the child demonstrated. Try to define the triggers for anger and outbursts, e.g. high-pitched noise, a previous activity

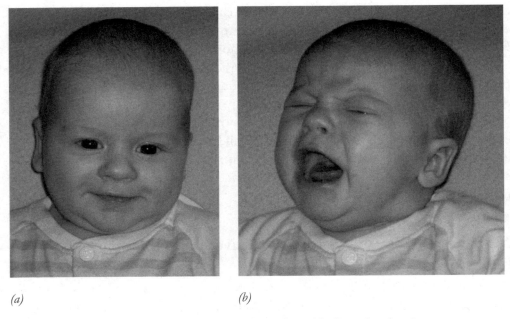

(a)   (b)

Figure 8.3a and b Children with Regulation Disorders may quickly change from happiness to extreme distress

during outside playtime, someone bumping into them, light touch, etc. Consider what preceded the tantrum/aggressive behavior as well as interactions that may have occurred with others.

Look at the four domains of regulation (sensory, motor, behavior and physiology) to see what areas might have contributed to the behavioral response, e.g. was the child tired, "wired" from the activity or setting, upset because of a change in routine?

Observing how the child responded will help to determine possible interventions. Did she yell, cringe, or punch someone? How long did the reaction last? Was the child eventually able to self-regulate or did the child need help?

Remember that many of the behaviors will be exactly how other children might respond in the same situation but for a child with RDSP, the behaviors may occur because of the child's heightened sensory responses, poor social interpretation or challenges with motor skills and the response may be more extreme. At times the child with RDSP will react with force with hard hits or squeezes and a loud voice either in play or during aggressive outbursts. To help the child realize what it feels like to be touched or hugged very hard, use different sensory materials. Show what happens and how it feels when play dough is squeezed softly or in different levels of strength. Use visual and physical clues to help her understand her own strength (e.g. lifting something heavy, pushing a wheelbarrow). When the child approaches adults with force and bangs into them, use a pillow between the child and the adult, while redirecting her to an alternate method of getting firm pressure and/or anger release. If a child is destroying objects, such as ripping a book, give the child a newspaper to rip or provide activities such as ripping up paper to be recycled, so she can use that activity when angry.

For children with RDSP, awareness of their own and others' voice levels and intonation is often lacking (although at other times they are highly alert to these factors). Ways to develop this could be in using tape recorders or videotape so the children can see and hear themselves. Some children have very loud sound outbursts but get very angry with others' "loud" voices.

It is necessary to differentiate and label calm and out-of-control behaviors. Help the child practice being calm and attentive when not angry. Compliment her on managing her behavior and staying calm when you observe these behaviors. Develop physical strategies for the child to use, e.g. holding on to her thumb, deep breathing. Develop a sequence of activities to help the child calm herself, such as cover her ears, get a soft toy, look at happy people.

Help the child to develop self-awareness of what is bothering her and help develop a script of the words needed to tell a parent and to tell others about her distress. Develop a visual picture for the child, e.g. the angry bugs that bother her. Social Stories™ can be used to review the acceptable responses (see Chapter 12 on Social Skills and the Resources section for information about Social Stories™).

For impulsive aggression, initially parents will have to help children to regulate their behavior but eventually children need to learn to take time out within themselves. The use of the turtle technique (Schneider and Robin 1973) may help children to have a process of either retreating or (for withdrawn uninvolved children) being involved in the event. This story can be adapted to a variety of situations and events, leading to interactive dialogue that is socially cued. For example, if a child is withdrawn you can point out that the turtle needs to get his head out to see the world; if the child is aggressive, the child needs to pull her head back in and get control.

The turtle story is as follows:

> Once upon a time there was a handsome young turtle. He was six years old and he had just started first grade. His name was Little Turtle. Little Turtle was very upset about going to school. He preferred to be at home with his baby brother and his mother. He didn't want to learn school things; he wanted to run outside and play with his friends, or color in his coloring book. It was too hard to try to write letters or copy them from the board. He wanted to play and giggle with friends – he even loved to fight with them. He didn't

like sharing. He didn't like listening to his teacher or having to stop making those wonderful loud fire engine noises he used to make with his mouth. It was too hard to remember not to fight or make noise. And it was just too hard not getting mad at all the things that made him mad.

Every day on his way to school he would say to himself that he would try his best not to get in trouble that day. But, despite that, every day he would get mad at somebody and fight, or he would get mad because he made a mistake and would rip up his papers. So he always would get into trouble, and after a few weeks, he just hated school. He began to feel like a "bad turtle." He went around for a long time feeling very, very bad.

One day when he was feeling his worst, he met the biggest, oldest tortoise in his town. He was a wise old turtle, who was 200 years old and as big as a house. Little Turtle spoke to him in a very timid voice because he was very afraid of him. But the old tortoise was as kind as he was big and was very eager to help him. "Hey there," he said in his big bellowing voice. "I'll tell you a secret. Don't you realize you are carrying the answer to your problem around with you?" Little Turtle didn't know what he was talking about. "Your shell – your shell!" he shouted. "That's why you have a shell. You can hide in your shell whenever you get that feeling inside of you that tells you that you are angry. When you are in your shell, you can have a moment to rest and figure out what to do about it. So next time you get angry, just go into your shell." Little Turtle liked the idea, and he was very eager to try his new secret in school.

The next day came and he again made a mistake on his nice clean paper. He started to feel that old angry feeling again and was about to lose his temper, when suddenly he remembered what the old tortoise had said. He pulled in his arms, legs and head, quick as a wink, and rested until he knew what to do. He was delighted to find it so nice and comfortable in his shell where no one could bother him. When he came out, he was surprised to find his teacher smiling at him. He told her he was angry about the mistake. She said she was very proud of him! He continued using his secret for the rest of the year. When he got his report card it was the best in the whole class. Everybody admired him and wondered what his magic secret was.

(Permission to reprint this story was kindly given by Dr. Robin, April 2006)

Code words for the child to use this technique could be as simple as "Turtle in now." As well, with this approach, relaxation techniques are taught and children are encouraged to close their eyes, place their chin on their chest, and pull their arms close to their body. The child is then taught to relax and tense her muscles. A critical component of this technique is to help the child to learn a problem-solving process with the goal being to have the child independently use the turtle process. This will then lead to the child receiving positive reinforcement for initiating appropriate responses to conflict.

Some responses to aggressive feelings, such as no touching, no physical violence, etc., need to be followed for all children. Think ahead of time how to manage the child's response to the consequence of such behaviors (e.g. being removed to her calming spot) since adult responses, when they are upset with the child's behavior, may be as disruptive as the child's initial behavior.

Adults can isolate themselves until they can calm themselves down, ignore some behaviors, and do not act on every behavior but instead concentrate on shifting critical ones, such as physically destructive behaviors. When the child acts indifferent or says "I don't care," adults need to calm themselves down before dealing with the behavior.

It is often helpful to use a cross modality to deal with the behaviors, for example if the child is verbally mocking, use touch and looks in response rather than talking to her (assuming she does not have tactile defensiveness). Define which senses the child responds to the most (both positively and negatively) and use the positive ones. This completes circles of communication without it being negatively interactive or the behaviors escalating.

When the child's capacity for sensory integration is at a low ebb (tired, sick, at the end of a high-activity day, anxious) adults need to respect the child's sensory tolerance. The adults must find and make small pockets of space and time where the child can feel safe and desensitize in small increments. Children with RDSP are often highly attuned to body language and gestures and how they are looked at by others. Discipline needs to be given in a calm, firm, soft voice.

At a crisis time when behaviors are deteriorating, the child may need to have an increased level of consistency for such aspects as bedtime. She may need even the fun times to be more regimented.

Although consistency and predictability in adult responses will best help the child to regain control, the child also needs to have some trial and error situations to learn. By defining what the behavioral expectations are, with less emphasis on what should not happen, this helps to direct her behaviors. Self-regulation for the child starts when the child has some opportunities to make mistakes and can cope with trying again.

Use of a "when – then" approach to discipline helps to define the behavioral consequences (framed in a positive way) for the child, for example "When you pick up your toys then we can go to the park." It also reminds the child of the needed sequence of behavior. This approach can also be used to show the cause and effect of the behavior. "Mom feels sad because…", "The boy is laughing because…"

Some suggestions frequently provided for helping children to manage their behavior do not work very well for the child with RDSP. For instance, ignoring behavior as a response may or may not work. Children may just increase their intensity of behavior. Removal from the situation may help the child to calm. A child-centered approach, such as saying, "I can see you are upset", "That must be difficult", may escalate the behavior. There is a need to set limits immediately so the child's behavior does not escalate.

Management strategies to help toddlers and young children self-calm

As an adult interacting with a child with RDSP, the ultimate goal is to help the child learn how to use self-calming techniques when she is upset. Just as most babies learn to suck their thumbs to self-soothe, so toddler, preschool and school-age children can learn methods to calm themselves. However, it may take a lot longer to help children with RDSP to learn these skills and they may need support and antici-pation of events and outcomes for far longer than other children. Being predictive of what may upset the child is important. Look for clues that the child is getting upset – changes in breathing, mottling on the chest and neck, flushed face and ears, jerky movements. Be aware of other stressors in the child's life so an adult can modify what the child has to cope with on a daily basis.

The child with RDSP may demonstrate affective storms (rage attacks). One moment the child may be calm and then explosive with very little lead-up. Remove the child from the environment until she is calm. Some adults find they have to hold the child; others have used placing the child between pillows (head out), or under a heavy blanket to help the child to calm down. Ensure that someone is supervising the child at all times during these interventions.

The adult can help provide an environment that will help the child to be able to use self-calming strategies (see Figure 8.4). Spending quiet time in their room, sitting in a beanbag chair, listening to music, use of a weighted vest for exciting, over-stimulating times – all are approaches that older children can learn to initiate themselves.

Other approaches such as relaxation strategies may need an adult to lead the process. The child may need to have visual pictures of which body part to relax and also a ball to squeeze rather than just trying to squeeze and relax specific muscles. Nightly reading of a story that has a lot of repetition and is about relaxation or sleep (see Resources section) may help with bedtime routines.

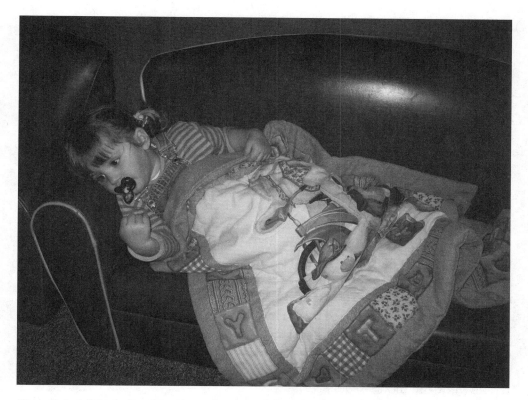

Figure 8.4 A "blankey" and soother are favorites to help with self-calming

Night time may be an especially difficult transition time for children who have difficulty self-calming. To decrease night terrors, put the child to bed earlier than usual before the child becomes really exhausted. Make sure the child is safe because sometimes, in her sleep state, she throw things or gets violent. Give a bath before dinner since for some children the bath routine energizes them.

Develop simple verbal phrases such as "Give me five." The child will need to be taught that this means eyes looking, ears listening, mouth quiet, hands folded, and sitting up. A picture of a hand and these words on it can reinforce the request. This eliminates lights out or clapping hands, bell, etc., to get attention since the child may find these noises irritating. Cue sentences such as "You need to get back in control", "Can you manage your behavior or do you need an adult to help?", "Make a smart choice" help children recognize that they have control over their own behaviour and cue them to stop or change their responses.

Use of reward systems and star charts may help reinforce desired behaviors and the child's capacity to manage her own behavior. (See Chapter 10.)

Help the child to recognize that at times everyone needs to take time away to calm down. Define a spot in the house that each family member uses for self-calming. This models for the child how and where one can gain control over one's behavior. The child's bedroom may not be the best spot for self-calming since it is primarily for sleep. Get the child to help select a spot where she feels comfortable.

Management strategies for under-reactive emotional behaviors

While aggressive and reactive emotional responses are most obviously problematic for the child and the people around her, the child who withdraws, does not become involved or retreats from involvement is demonstrating behaviors that may be equally concerning. While these children are seldom viewed as having behavior problems, because they do not easily engage in social interactions, their repertoire of social language and skills may be decreased. They may not move or engage in physical activities as much as their peers and their muscles become weaker. They may require more intense touch, smells or sounds to attend to an event. They may appear to not feel pain. Heightened input and high-interest activities need to be used to engage these children in participating.

Combining one or more sensory inputs with verbal or visual input helps the child receive input in at least one of these senses. For instance, when teaching a multistep activity, hand-over-hand may help increase the child's learning speed and retention of the motor sequence.

Analyze games and activities for the variety of senses that are required. Choose games and activities that have a sensory component, such as Body Boggle where body movement and positioning is a large component or Hungry Hippo where sound and movement of the game parts increases awareness. Games that require two or more participants to be involved help the child to remain alert and encourage development of social skills.

Adults can alert the child to differences in reaction by exaggerating their own emotions and actions and varying the loudness and tone of their voice to get the child's attention.

Teaching children jokes provides them with an age-appropriate skill and helps alert them to language. However, often an explanation of why the joke is funny is needed. Make humor personal by watching comedy films and making family films of a Silly Day or a Backwards Day.

Comment on smells and feeling textures and relate them to personal feelings, for example "I love the smell of popcorn because it makes me think of movies I have enjoyed", "That fleecy blanket reminds me of when you were a teeny tiny baby."

Specifically teach safety behaviors about fire, electrical outlets, and sharp objects.

Management strategies to decrease perseverative behaviors

Many parents wonder if the perseverative behaviors their child displays are just a phase or if they are obsessive. The behaviors often make the child stand out as different within their peer group or in public settings. Often a decision has to be made of which battles to fight – whether safety issues are involved or whether the child's behaviour will result in scape-goating or ridicule. It is useful to know that many of the behaviors change or fade away over time.

Focusing on one topic or activity is less anxiety provoking for the children. Observe when the child is most often involved in using perseverative behaviors. Introduce relaxation techniques and use of music, movement and deep pressure to help self-calm if it appears she is feeling anxious. Obsessive thoughts and ritual behaviors are often linked to a bigger picture (e.g. if a family has a new baby in the house). The child may feel out of control of her regular routine and what she can expect. The repetitive actions have meaning to the child and appear to soothe her (see Figure 8.5).

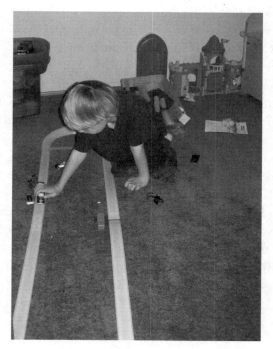

Figure 8.5 Some children use repetitive behaviors as a self-calming mechanism when they are anxious or stressed

If adults promote the "obsession" of the child then she may become even more stuck on that behavior. There is a need to limit the activity by offering the child different ideas, an expansion of the positive parts and shifting of the repetitive aspects. Offer the child different approaches, language, ideas around the repetitive behaviors; for example, if the child will only wear blue clothing, expand her thinking to all the shades of blue, how the blue sky changes at sunset and the shades of color in the blue sea. Paint pictures using these ideas. This use of thematic expansion – expanding the child's single focus ideas and fitting her ideas into other ideas (e.g. take a fascination with trains and teach about engines, trips to different places, food from other countries that are transported by trains) – helps deflect and alter the perseverative behaviors.

Greenspan and Weider (1998) use creative approaches (described in their book *The Child With Special Needs*) that can help shift the child's responses and perceptions as she is involved in repetitive play/behaviors. Start where the child is physically and emotionally at within her play behaviors and then gradually introduce a difference by your own behavioral interactions. (Also see Floor Time website resource for additional information.)

Many adults have found that if it is not disruptive to the child's life or a safety issue, then they might as well go along with the behavior (e.g. wanting to wear the same dancing outfit to school every day). Concerns over social implications with other children teasing or bullying the child as they get older indicate a need for monitoring social interactions. If the obsessive behaviors also interfere with play, school work, or home tasks then this is a problem that needs to be addressed. As the child gets older she will be more responsive to social norms. At that point she may be motivated to seek help to solve problems that her sensory needs create that may have contributed to the perseverative behaviors.

Children with RDSP are often hyper-vigilant about the behaviors of others. They often focus on the "truth" or a "promise" and have a very black-and-white perception of the social world. Do not make promises to the children since they will seldom forget this type of statement and will not accept circumstances that might require a shift from the original promise. Practice responses with the child about events that may not be "fair", such as one child getting more turns than another.

Management strategies to create routines

Especially during the preschool years, there are two additional consistent challenges in the affective organization areas of development that occur with children with RDSP. One is the *inflexibility* that the children demonstrate in the face of changing family, school or community activities, and the other is difficulty *coping with transitions* in situations such as changing from one activity to another, from one situation to another, or from one adult or playmate to another.

Routines help to give children with RDSP a sense of predictability in at least some aspects of their lives. These children may need to have their routines maintained for most of their childhood so many of these suggestions may need to be continued on into school years. While this may appear to encourage inflexibility and rigidity in behaviors, the use of routines within the family and community will decrease arguments and lessen anxiety for the children.

For non-reading children, develop a picture sequence of the events that will happen throughout the day. Drawings can be used or take pictures of the child doing the activities, laminate them and put Velcro on the back. These pictures are now available to arrange on a board with Velcro tabs, in the sequence of events that will occur on any specific day.

Develop predictable routines within the home related to times when struggles are most likely to occur, such as bedtime, morning routines and mealtimes. Ask ahead about family routines when visiting friends and extended family, so a description can be made to the child of what will likely happen at the new house. Plan ahead and give realistic choices of what children can do during family or group activities (such as shopping in a noisy mall) that are too stimulating or aversive for them (e.g. they get to play in the ball room at the end, they can wear their walkman, they can ride in the cart).

Once established, the routines may be difficult to change. If change is necessary introduce small changes over time; for example, if Dad is going to read the bedtime story, start with him reading part of it and Mom finishing the story for several nights.

Be spontaneous in times when as an adult you do not have to respond to societal pressure – the child needs to cope with some variety too and everyone deserves to have flexible times together.

Management strategies to help with transitions

We often talk about attachment of a child. Attachment means that the parents have bonded to the child as well as the child to the parent.

When the child goes into the world from a secure base (the parent) she will move from the parent and be able to explore and develop new skills. When the child is distressed, she will go to the secure base for the parent to help with calming. Children with RDSP often need an adult to initiate help in learning self-calming skills for a longer period of time than other children.

The child with RDSP may exhibit social anxiety when new things happen or do not go well or there is not a familiar adult to reassure her. This is often precipitated at times of transition. Her behavior may appear as aggression, crying, rejection of support or withdrawal.

When the child is distressed at school or in community activities, she will look for a secure base. Unlike at home, at school or in the community this secure base may not be available. When there are no supports, it is harder for the child's own impulse controls to work. While it is not easy to modify the educational or community systems, it is important to address the instructional approach and environmental needs to allow for development of the secure base for the child. One solution is for the child to have a defined ally with whom she feels comfortable, to help with transitions.

Transitions from activity to activity and from place to place may be difficult. The child may have problems moving from one thought to another, which may result in repetitive thoughts and sayings that help the child to feel secure when involved with an unfamiliar activity.

There are a number of predictable but critical periods of transition throughout the life of a child. The ability to walk and talk for the toddler brings both more independence and challenges. Beginning preschool introduces variety and other people, rules and restraints to the child. Entering kindergarten increases the contact with a larger number of children, a more structured environment and input from a variety of adults. At the beginning of intermediate grades, both cognitive, academic and social expectations increase as the child is expected to think at a more abstract level and become more independent and interactive in social interactions. The end of elementary school years brings more complex social interactions, independence and more advanced critical thinking.

If adults are alert to these transition times they can help the child to be proactive in how to manage the changes. Helping the child with RDSP to know the whole sequence of the upcoming activity may decrease her anxiety and resistance. For activities that are similar in sequence each time, have pictures to show the sequence of the activities. For new activities that will happen in the future, take the child ahead of time to see/do the new activity on her own before the activity is integrated into the sequence (e.g. if going to a new babysitter after preschool, visit ahead of time to see the toys and meet the person). The child may need to have a familiar transitional object (e.g. a teddy, toy train or blanket) between spending time with one adult and another or changing from one activity to another.

The use of timers or a countdown for leaving a place, and defining the sequence preceding the time to leave, is useful to give the child time to adjust. Take a repetitive thought or saying and lead it into another expressed thought, comment or activity; for example, "I want to go out, I want to go out, I want to go out…" and the parent says, "I want to go out and we will get Benjamin at school" which helps direct the child's thinking beyond the immediate activity.

Collect a series of transitional activities that can be completed in a brief time. A stacking toy for young children, a small puzzle with few pieces, a Lego set that has only a few pieces, a small book, a transformer toy, allows the child to do a short interim activity before going on to the next longer activity.

Anticipating changes is essential. Introduce new things gradually (e.g. if furniture in the home is moved, do a few pieces of furniture at a time). It is especially important to plan ahead for institutional transitions (see Chapter 11 on preparing the child with Regulation Disorders for school). Be physically available for the child at times of known transitions institutional and otherwise (e.g. when the child comes out of the preschool classroom, at bedtime, when turning off a video for supper).

Summary

- A child's ability to regulate her moods and feelings is considered one indicator of development of mature behavioral responses. Emotions have "twin tasks" of regulating affect in response to others and the environment, and being regulated by oneself. The dimensions that affect emotional responses are the intensity of emotion, the person's threshold of response, and their windows of tolerance to emotions.

- Development of a secure attachment with a positive caretaker helps a child to organize her emotions more effectively. While routines serve a useful purpose in helping lessen anxiety and increasing attention and organization in the child with RDSP, children with perseverative behaviors and underactive emotional responses need help in shifting these responses. Responses to transitions also often increase the intensity of emotional responses and coping strategies need to be developed.

- Self-regulation, self-awareness, and self-monitoring in affected areas contribute to positive social interactions within the home, school and community. Children with RDSP often need support in managing their emotional responses for far longer than their peers.

Chapter 9

BEHAVIORAL ORGANIZATION AND PROCESSING – ATTENTION REGULATION

Attention to a task requires both the ability to establish initial focus and to sustain attention until the task is completed. A newborn baby demonstrates an orienting system that allows the babsy to focus on his caregiver and food source. The baby rapidly becomes responsive to novelty, to facial expressions of others and to sounds and movement. Textures and shape become as important as color and pattern as the baby begins to expand his sensory world. By the end of the first year a more prolonged and complex level of attention has developed, although infants are still distracted by novelty. Older children are more distracted by events in their environment or, once their language develops, labeling and the meaning of words.

It is easy to see why a child with Regulation Disorders of Sensory Processing (RDSP) with prominent attention control difficulties would resemble a child with Attention Deficit Hyperactivity Disorder (ADHD). The features of impulsiveness and stimulus-seeking are common to both these disorders. In clinical practice, it may take a long time to differentiate between these two conditions. Therefore, parents should insist that their child be seen on several occasions when a diagnosis is in doubt. Evaluation by a multidisciplinary team also helps clarify the diagnosis.

A number of observations need to be made to exclude the differential diagnosis. Control requiring thoughtful responses may be more difficult for children with ADHD as compared to children with RDSP. Pervasiveness of behaviors (behaviors that occur in multiple settings), a feature that must be present to diagnose ADHD, may be irrelevant in RDSP. A common confusing feature is that while both these conditions start in the early years, in the case of ADHD, parents most often describe the hyperactivity as beginning when the child became mobile, while parents of children with RDSP describe a history of fussy, difficult-to-soothe infants who early on develop high activity and attention difficulties.

Management strategies to help infants and toddlers attend

"Joint attention" – the ability to attend to another object and still attend to the caregiver – is developed over time. Adults can help to gradually increase an infant and toddler's attention for interactions and involvement in activities. Initially a baby attends to either an object (e.g. a crib toy) or its mother or father. As the child's ability to attend increases, a third object can be introduced while the parent is playing with the baby. At two years old a child should be able to attend for two to three minutes on a task (see Figures 9.1a and b).

When infants demonstrate inattention to tasks such as feeding, make the room where they are fed as neutral as possible – eliminate bright lights, multicolored pictures or loud high-pitched musical toys and bright clothes while holding the child. Instead, quiet music, and such considerations as single colored clothes for the mother, may help direct the infant to the task at hand.

Linking toys where the adult does one piece and the child does another to make the whole (e.g. pop-it beads, stacking toys) help develop both reciprocal interactions and attention.

Use brief playtimes with the infant to extend his attention to toys or activities. Present one toy and help the child to learn the many aspects of the toy (movement, shape, texture, sound, etc.).

If an infant gets highly excited and distracted, remove him from the event until he is calm. Use a soft calm voice, and gently hold or rock to decrease excessive movement.

Limit television watching. (Yes, some adults use the TV as a soother for their infant or toddler!) While the child may sustain attention for the children's shows, they are one-dimensional, have frequent changes in topic and short visual input and do not encourage sustained attention.

For children with low sensory responses, read books that have a high visual and sensory appeal (talking books, "feely" books). Select toys that have multiple uses and sensory input. Obtaining toys from suppliers that produce toys specifically for children with sensory needs will ensure a high quality of toy at an appropriate developmental level (see resources section).

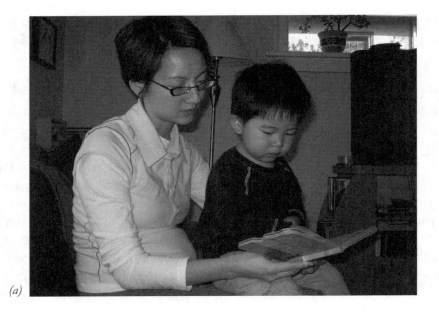

(a)

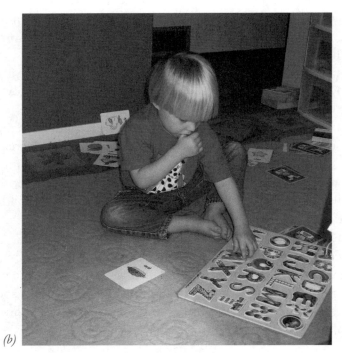

(b)

Figures 9.1a and b Ensuring that books and toys are at the appropriate developmental level will help the child to attend

Management strategies to increase attention in preschool and school-age children

Many of the tasks that a child will encounter in preschool and school settings require sustained attention, with the amount of time the child is expected to attend increasing as the child gets older.

If the child has difficulty with maintaining attention to a task, consider if the activity is at a developmental level that a child of this age would ordinarily be expected to complete. There are a number of excellent paperback books that outline developmental skills at ages from birth upwards (see Resources section).

Analyze the individual activity to consider how much and what kind of skills (perceptual, cognitive, motor/movement) the task requires. Consider each aspect of the skill. This includes:

- motor movement – gross motor or fine motor or both, fast or slow speed

- perceptual skills – visual, kinesthetic, proprioception, auditory

- cognition – knowledge base, memory requirements, abstract or concrete thinking, imitation and language requirements.

Break down the activity into component parts if the child is having difficulty and then build up the skill, doing each section step by step.

Completion may require several times of working on the task. Use a "goal, plan, do, check" approach (see information in Chapter 6 on motor responses and CanChild website in Resources section) to help the child succeed at tasks and to continue activities through to completion.

Decrease distractions within the learning environment – whether the task is learning to put on socks or drawing a circle. Do not have the television or computer on, or toys in sight or available, when attempting to encourage skills such as staying at the dinner table or getting ready to go outside. However, do have small toys available when the child has to wait for periods of time in public situations (e.g. a restaurant, in a lineup, at the doctor's). By selecting toys that are fun and educational, these times when children are frequently grumpy and inattentive have the potential to become more positive and to help the child learn to both attend and wait.

Plan each day to include social, sensory and motor activities either within the family activities or during play with other children. Move from familiar activities to short times of experiencing new activities. Ensure that movement and fun activities are interspersed between more specific sit-down learning/fine motor activities.

Additional suggestions for how to help the child attend are available in books written for parents and teachers of children with ADHD (see Resources section).

Summary

- The ability to attend to an activity is an important developmental task that contributes to skill attainment in self-care, academic and leisure activities.

- Some children with RDSP have difficulty attending and may be mistakenly diagnosed as having ADHD. Children with RDSP have the capacity for effortful control and demonstrate less pervasiveness of inattention than children with ADHD. A structured environment and a gradual increase in the length of attention required for tasks, as well as other suggestions used to help children who *do* have ADHD to manage their inattention, can assist to increase behavioral organization and processing in the areas of attention. As the child grows, it is not unusual to see RDSP and ADHD coexisting.

Chapter 10

REGULATION OF BEHAVIOR

While many of the extreme behaviors that children with Regulation Disorders of Sensory Processing (RDSP) exhibit can be attributed to their unique processing of sensory input, they also will have behaviors that are responsive to their environment, interactions with peers and siblings and driven by their own temperament. Parents therefore will need to have skills in helping deal with these behaviors – and these skills are similar to the parenting skills needed in responding to and guiding any child.

Star charts to encourage appropriate behaviors

Development of a reward system to shift problematic behaviors is a useful approach. A reward chart is visual, immediate, and helps a child develop a capacity to manage her own behaviors. The main objective of a reward system is to *catch the child being good*! Star charts use the principles of operant conditioning – rewards given for appropriate behaviors. They are used to help the child internalize values and reasons for appropriate behaviors. The rewards should not be an end in themselves and focus on material gain, but should focus on aspects that are usually more valued by the child such as time with her parent/caregiver/peers to do something special such as games with siblings, or small events such as making popcorn together. There are a number of principles to follow in the development of an effective star chart:

- Select only three or four behaviors and always have one behavior that the child can always attain. Define, using positive wording, exactly what the behavior will look like (e.g. "I will use my words when angry" rather than "No hitting when angry"; "Hang my clothes on the hooks" rather than "Don't leave my clothes on the floor").

- For young children under six years of age, make sure that the day is divided into short periods of time (30-minute time frames maximum) to gain stars frequently in each of the behavior areas. Older children continue to need frequent reinforcement (e.g. morning, noon, after school, supper, bedtime) for getting the earned stars. Do not take away tokens (stars, pennies, bingo dots, pom-poms) that have been earned.

- Children will inevitably grow bored with a star chart. Be prepared to vary the method, using stamps, stickers, cubes, pennies, and bingo dots. Use different sizes of stars – small ones for a small reward, big ones for a big reward to be gained after attaining incrementally more correct behaviors.

- Make sure the chips, stars or markers are kept in a secure place so children do not reward themselves when parents are not looking. Hang the star chart in a very visible area so all family members can see how well the child is doing in managing her behavior and compliment the child on her success.

Developing a reward system

Having a variety of predetermined rewards that have high interest but little cost is useful. This will eliminate negotiating by the child or a feeling by the adult that the child is being "bought" to show appropriate behavior. Some of the categories and possible rewards that other parents have used are listed below. Many are items that are usually reserved for treats, and that is what they are – treats for positive behavior rather than "a given."

Food

- Special main course meal: Select from a predetermined list of favorites, e.g. pizza, fish and chips.

- Drink: Chocolate milk, fruit punch, fizzy fruit juice, yogurt drink.

- Dessert: Choice of a bakery cookie, ice-cream, cake, pie.

- Snack food: Raisin boxes, popcorn or nuts (if age appropriate – do not give if under five or if child has chewing and swallowing difficulties; check for allergies), chips, sesame snaps, dried fruit, fruit leather, fruit or pudding cups, fruit juice Popsicles.

Toys and games

(Identify the specific games by name – select age-appropriate games for the child, not based on the interests of other family members.) Board games, card games, action people, construction toys, video games, computer games, puppets.

Books

(Identify the names of the books on a list. Many books and some tapes can be loaned from local libraries.) Find books with a read-along tape, or use comics, magazines, learn to draw books.

Arts and crafts

Drawing, painting, play dough, plasticine, simple woodworking, model making, large-bead jewellery making.

Activities and sports

(Select age-appropriate sports/activities.) Bowling, riding a bike, hiking, shooting baskets, playing baseball, table tennis/ping pong, soccer, fishing, skateboarding, playground equipment, jump rope, street/floor hockey, table hockey, camping, ice skating, ball games.

Music activities

Playing real or home-made instruments (e.g. a comb and wax paper), listening to tapes and compact discs (CDs), use of a walkman radio, dancing to music for fun.

Outings and activities

Local parks and playgrounds, community center for Moms/Dads and tots or open gym (if child can tolerate the noise), amusement park, movie, child-friendly restaurant, aquarium, outdoor concerts, nature park.

Special one-to-one time with parent or other adult

Helping a parent with simple cooking (pizza toppings) or fun cooking (cut-out cookies), reading together, playing a game together, going on a treasure hunt.

Timeout

When a child with RDSP has a tantrum or other emotional crisis, how can timeout be used? Point out that everyone needs time to calm down. If a child can see the time away as purposeful and not negative – as a time to get control and not as a punishment – then they are more likely to respond without fuss. The purpose of calming down needs to be clearly defined and the parents serious and consistent about its use. During a time that the child is calm, role-play and explain the purpose of timeout. Children often respond better to the phrase "calming down" rather than "timeout." Select a calming chair/area. Each family member can have a calming method – music, reading the paper, a bath. The child can have a calming method, such as coloring, to do within their own calming area. Length of timeouts should be no more than a minute per year of age up to age five, and no longer than ten minutes in total for any child.

Consistency and inconsistency

At times parents/caregivers/educators will be inconsistent in their behaviors. It is important to explain why the changes have happened, and to acknowledge mistakes if that is what caused a change or inconsistency. This can help children learn about how to negotiate when mistakes are made. As well they can learn about authenticity and trust within family relationships which will contribute to an ability to form relationships outside the home. Children are often insightful about their own reactions and behaviors. They need to be encouraged to realize that they are capable of participating in solving problems. When problems related to inconsistency or other reasons arise, adults need to ask the child "How can we solve this problem?" and use a problem-solving approach:

1. Name the problem.

2. Think of at least three ways to solve the problem.

3. Pick one solution that could make the problem better.

4. Is it safe? Is it fair? How will it make people feel? Will it work?

4. Try it – if it doesn't work, try one of the other solutions.

Management strategies for specific events within the home and community

There are a number of situations and events within homes and communities that parents have found create more difficulty for their child with RDSP than for other children. The following information provides suggestions for management of behaviors in the areas that parents have suggested are particularly problematic.

Community needs

Unpredictable and loud noise or excessive activity often occur in the community and cultural activities to which parents may want to introduce their child. By choosing community activities where parents and children are together (e.g. Moms and Tots gym, art or dance for parents and children, woodworking or craft activities sponsored by businesses in the community), the child's responses can be monitored and help given to either calm the child or encourage the child to become more involved during the activities. Plan to go for shorter periods of time than an entire production at a children's theater or other structured event. Reserve seats from which there is an easy exit. Seek out plays and music events etc. that are held in the outdoors where children can move about or stand at the back of the area. Wait until the orchestra has finished tuning their instruments before entering musical events.

When adults change their usual routes when walking or driving throughout the community with a child with RDSP, the child may become upset. Change the routes a bit at a time, to encourage flexibility. Tell the child ahead of time about the plan to drive or walk one block differently this time. For older children show on a map the driving or walking route and encourage them to look at the map when traveling. Print out their own map on a computer map-maker program.

Medical and dental needs

The extreme behavioral and sensory responses of a child with RDSP often mean that specialized healthcare professionals need to be found. The location of doctors and dentists who are used to working with children with resistant and/or aggressive behaviors is essential. Be prepared to educate the family's general practitioner, community health nurse and dentist about RDSP so they understand why a referral to a specialist or a colleague who has special skills with children may be requested.

- Visit the medical office with the child and meet the health practitioner before going for an appointment when the practitioner examines the child.

- Role-play the activities that may happen before going to the office.

- Create a Social Story™ related to what the child can expect at the dentist or doctor's office. Review the story before arriving at the office.

- Tell the truth – that an inoculation will hurt a bit, that there will be strange smells at the dentist.

- When taking the child to the dentist for cleaning or repair ask for sedatives for the child if her reaction is extreme to these events.

Leaving the house

The transition of leaving the familiar environment of home to go to an unknown or more stimulating environment may result in problems for a child with RDSP. If the child's behavior deteriorates when leaving home, warn the child in plenty of time that everyone will be leaving. Describe the sequence of what the family will be doing. Get the child to help with some task of leaving, such as carrying the shopping bags. Have a visual picture reminder by the door related to what is needed when leaving the house, for example snack, jackets, boots, car toys, Mom's purse, etc. This will also help children to think in an organized fashion in their own lives. Children function at their own pace – determine how slow the child moves and allow enough time. Warn the child of the time left. Use a visual timer to indicate the passage of time. Include a "leaving the house on time" item on the child's star chart if this is a recurrent problem.

Behavior in the car

If a child refuses to get into a car seat, keep her hands busy while putting the child in the car seat by letting her hold a book to read or eat cereal from a small container. Many children do not like the restraints of seatbelts, which of course must be worn (see Figure 10.1). Make sure they are wearing their most comfortable clothes so they do not feel restrained by clothing as well. Use of a car video may help the child to focus on something pleasurable that has only one area to focus on, as you drive along. If yelling or fighting occurs with a sibling in the car, provide a walkman with

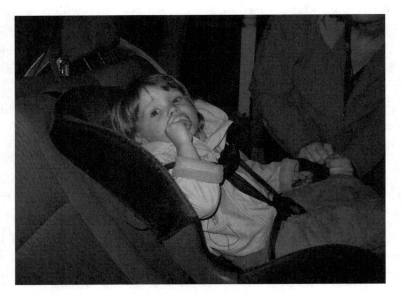

Figure 10.1 The closed environment, seatbelt restraints and noise and movement of a car may create distress for the child with Regulation Disorders

music tapes or a read-and-listen book. Have a container of toys for each child to use. Use a large tall pillow to separate children in the back seat.

Some children find the sway of a car or the movement of the outside objects going by very upsetting. Try using earphones and a music recording as distraction, encourage napping while in the car, and help the child to learn to look straight ahead rather than turning her own head about. Use a window screen to decrease flickering light or visual awareness of objects racing by. Be prepared to pull over to the side of the road until the child calms down if she becomes very upset while in a moving car.

Public transit

Public transit, with the noise, stops and starts, people entering and exiting and sur-rounding talk and laughter, can be a very aversive environment for a child with RDSP. However, increasingly families are using public transit for both environ-mental and economic reasons. Strategic selection of where the adult and child sit can offset some of the possible problems. On city buses, sit so that the child is in the window seat and is not touched by other adults or children. Sit near the front or the doors so there is no need to walk by numerous people in or out of the bus and so an easy exit can be made if the child becomes upset. On a plane, try to book the bulkhead seat or the window seats. Sit in smoke-free areas if these exist, especially if the child is sensitive to smells.

Become familiar with the routes and the drivers and try to avoid the drivers who joke and get the whole bus laughing or who are loud or talkative to passengers, especially if the child is sensitive to noise. If carrying a baby, make minimal responses to individuals who get up close to the baby and want to engage in a con-versation about the child.

A sense of hurrying when using public transit often feels inevitable. Take as much time as needed when getting strollers off and on the bus. If the adult becomes agitated, the child may also get upset.

Ensure that the physiological needs of the child are met before boarding public transit. Dress the child in layered clothing since she may become over-heated in buses. Use the toilet before travel and take a small snack for eating while on the vehicle. Carry along a bag of small toys, coloring materials, small puzzles to enter-tain the child if traveling by bus, train, ferry or plane.

For the child and the adult's safety, use a child harness when boarding in areas where there are many pedestrians, such as in train or subway stations. Try not to travel alone. A traveling companion can help avoid or manage many of the situa-tions discussed above.

Highly stimulating events – birthday parties, seasonal events

Events which adults hope their children will most enjoy often create the most distress. Change of routine, noise, bright lights, flash bulbs, visiting relatives and neighbors, different foods, all are possible contributions to negative responses in a child with RDSP. Considering the sensory, motor and behavioral responses of the child with RDSP and planning for these events with these aspects in mind may increase the positive outcome.

Try to provide for hunger, sleep and elimination needs ahead of time since these needs may precipitate troublesome behaviors or result in emotional dys-regulation when combined with a stimulating event. Decide which adult will give instructions, requests and directions. Limit the number of visiting relatives during any family event.

Monitor the location of children's parties to which the child has been invited (e.g. going to McDonald's play ball room may be too stimulating when there are ten other children). Ask the hosting parent if an adult familiar to the child can attend the party to monitor the responses of the child to the crowd, the activities and the excitement. This will also provide a resource to help the child calm down if neces-sary. An ideal party is with a small number of children – one or two children with whom the child can get along. Limit the gifts and emphasize adult supervised games. Keep the time frame short.

Assess ahead of time if the child can tolerate the singing of Happy Birthday. Some children get very upset with discordant singing. See if a recorded Happy Birthday song could be used.

Arrange activities where all the children can do their own thing, such as swimming pool parties, rather than structured games. Loud noises and high activity levels (e.g. ball room, tag games) are often too stimulating. When the child gets stressed there is often an increase in her reactions and sensitivities.

Restaurant meals

Parents and other family members want the flexibility of enjoying a family meal in a restaurant from time to time. To help the child with RDSP to accept and enjoy these events, select a child-friendly restaurant on a week day so there will be less noise and fewer people. Go to the restaurant before the day of the expected meal. Sit at the table and have a soft drink. At home, role-play restaurant behaviors and responses. Include having the "waiter" ask the family for food choices, having to wait for the food, etc. Create a Social Story™ to review behaviors and sequences. Take the story to the restaurant to review it at the beginning of the event. Take a bag of toys, crayons and books to entertain the child while waiting for service at a restaurant. Ask for a table that enables an easy exit if that becomes necessary.

Check to see if you can take favorite foods to be heated in the restaurant microwave if that is necessary to avoid an issue over the type of food the child will eat. Have dessert such as a takeout ice-cream cone on the way home rather than extending the time in the restaurant to include eating a dessert.

Home responsibilities

Sometimes it seems more bother than it is worth to encourage highly reactive or low-response children to participate in household activities. However, it has been shown that one aspect contributing to resiliency in children is for them to assume some age-appropriate responsibilities within their own home. As well, recognition as a contributing family member helps increase a child's self-esteem. To ensure cooperation and decrease struggles, determine age-appropriate household tasks for each child. Have a picture of what the child's room should look like when it is clean and when it is not clean so the child can see the criteria. To streamline tasks, use specific baskets for clothes and toys to decrease possible problems with motor skills or figure-ground and spatial relations perception. Make doing the task worthwhile in the child's mind. Include at least one home responsibility on the reward star chart. For children who can read, have a short list of the chores in the sequence they need to be done. For those who can not yet read, have a sequence of pictures.

Summary

- Development of a behavioral management plan to deal with the behavioral responses of children with RDSP will help increase their self-regulation and lessen anger and distress among the adults who work and play with and love them. Many of the behavioral responses are similar to those of any regular child, but are more extreme and intense and prolonged than their peers.

- Behavioral management strategies suggested for use with regular children, such as use of star charts, reward systems and a calm-down time, can also be effective with children with RDSP, although the approaches may need some alterations to address the unique sensory and motor responses of the child. Consistency and routine help to decrease anxiety and promote a positive response from the child.

- A proactive analytic approach to special events such as birthday parties, traveling on public transportation, or going for doctor or dentist visits allows the adult to circumvent some of the inevitable responses that may occur with a child with RDSP.

Part Three

THE IMPACT OF
REGULATION
DISORDERS

Chapter 11

THE SCHOOL SYSTEM
AND THE CHILD WITH
REGULATION DISORDERS

When a child with Regulation Disorders of Sensory Processing (RDSP) goes to school it is a transition for both the child and the family. There needs to be emotional preparedness, awareness of the physical environment and acceptance by the educators of the milieu and assistance that the child may need.

A diagnosis defining the child as having RDSP is essential to help shift the perception of the child as oppositional and willful and of the parents as being incompetent and causing the problem.

For children with Regulation Disorders of Sensory Processing (RDSP), there may be a delay or omission of the usual stages of development of emotional maturity. Maturity will come for the child, but the child may still need adults giving concrete guidance at home and in the community and providing this scaffolding for a longer period than for other children who do not have RDSP.

Before the child enters preschool or kindergarten

Education of the educators is very important, both about RDSP and the implications of the disorder. Sharing information with educators about strategies such as behavioral management and specific approaches such as Social Stories™ and responses to sensory reactions can help the child both at home and in the school.

Teachers, aides and principals need to be open to listening to the parents as they describe the specific needs, reactions and interventions that have worked with their child.

If parents and educators work together, effective solutions can be developed. Parents have often been blamed for inadequate parenting skills by family, friends and the community because of their child's responses and behaviors. They do not need blaming repeated within the school setting.

Professional development days need to include information about classroom management strategies for children with RDSP. Aides assigned to the child need specific information about the child and for children with RDSP in general.

Guidelines need to be developed for writing Individual Education Plans/Programs (IEPs) for the children and their specific needs, as well as general needs, so they can include strategies to respond to such aspects as heightened sensory reactions.

Choosing an appropriate school

The neighborhood preschool/school may provide the perfect environment for the child with RDSP but it is important to investigate all of the educational possibilities and make a choice dependent on the specific needs of the individual child. Visit a number of preschools/schools before deciding on the appropriate one for the child.

For some children, an alternative school setting, such as the Montessori schooling approach allowing both exploration and learning at their own speed while also providing structure, is very effective. When making a choice of schools, consider that if the child is enrolled in a private school, there may be a different culture between home and school. Aspects such as the expected rules and social etiquette may be at odds and present either too much diversity or rigidity for the child. A "traditional school" may provide consistency and predictability but not be flexible enough to respond to the child's unique needs. As well, travel in school buses or for extended periods of time to get to an out-of-neighborhood school may create problems.

School uniforms, traditionally required by private schools, may present a problem. The child with RDSP may be reactive to the materials used (wool or synthetics) in the uniforms or to the ties and closed shoes that are often required. These tactile sensitivities could interfere with an early positive bonding to the school and teachers.

Develop links with parents who have had children in the preschool or kindergarten that is being considered and who know how the classroom is organized. At the end of the preschool year, try to access the use of supported childcare (educational assistants) to help with the transitions into the kindergarten school environment. Determine ahead of time, by talking with the principal, which of the teachers is reasonably flexible and willing to learn about the needs of the child.

If team teaching occurs (two teachers within a large class), the teacher who the child responds to the best should be his major teacher. This choice will need to occur several weeks after school starts in the fall, after the child has been integrated into the class.

Documentation by the parents of what management strategies are successful and what resources are needed is important. As well, each year, before the child enters the next grade, ask the teacher to write a report of strategies that have worked well in terms of classroom teaching and behavior management with the child. This report – teacher to teacher – can then be passed on to the next teacher. Ask the family doctor to write a letter supporting extra school staff assistance if this is considered necessary for the child.

Document the types of sensory responses that the child has and how he typically reacts. Anticipate what school activities and/or sensory input may precipitate behaviors within the child (e.g. lunchroom, gym, circle time). Develop a handbook for the teachers (and daycare and community workers) of critical events that may cause problems and provide possible problem-solving strategies; for example, when lining up at the door, let the child stand at the side. Write down the behavior management strategies that work well at home so there is documentation and consistency in expectation and manner of dealing with behaviors. Categorize management strategies so that it can be a ready reference for the teachers (e.g. managing temper outbursts, managing transitions, etc.). Teachers will need to know what situations they will need to work around and those that will need to be dealt with in a consistent manner. If Social Stories™ are being used to help the child to learn social skills and responses (or other life skills), provide a copy for the school and add to these stories as situations arise.

Investigation of availability and type of after-school care, if both parents are working, is also necessary. Minimizing changes of location and staff, and ensuring that staff will follow consistent practices with the child, are important considerations.

Parents need to develop an overview of the resources that are available in the school district and how to access them, for example special needs consultant, school counselor, psychologist, supported childcare, learning assistance teachers, speech and language therapists, and occupational therapists. During the early years of their child's education they may have need of one or more of these specialized staff and it helps to know ahead of time exactly who works in the district and their service mandate.

Assessing a classroom for a child with Regulation Disorders

When assessing the appropriateness of a classroom for a child with RDSP, it is suggested that the parent liaise with the principal, the school counselor or a special education consultant assigned to the school to discuss the following considerations.

1. How are individual learning differences accommodated?

2. What types of learning activities are used? Are learning tasks presented using a multisensory approach?

3. What is the length of each learning activity?

4. What is the ratio of one-to-one versus group work?

5. How much work is done in a circle versus non-circle?

6. What type of behavior management is used in the class?

7. What are the priorities in behavior management techniques?

8. Is a developmental basis used for the curriculum and behavior management?

9. Is there consistency in behavior rewards and consequences?

10. How are age-appropriate social skills encouraged?

11. Is there involvement of older children/other adults with the class?

12. Does the classroom have predictable routines?

13. Does the classroom allow parent participation?

14. What sort of parent/teacher communication is encouraged?

15. What types of assessments are used with the children?

16. What academic resource staff is available within the school?

17. Note the ratio of teachers to children, the staff knowledge about the needs of special needs children, and access to supported childcare, speech and language and occupational therapy in the preschool/school.

Educating the child with Regulation Disorders about school

Although most children learn to conform readily to the rules and regulations of preschool and school, the child with RDSP often has difficulty. Educating the child about what to expect during the school day is as important as educating him about the unspoken rules and regulations of school.

Prepare the child by setting up several visits for the child and parent before the beginning of school. Visit when there are no children and then when the class is in progress and there is more noise, confusion, announcements, etc. It will be easier for the child to tolerate this when a parent is there with the child for the first time. Tell the child what will be expected of him, rehearse responses, and answer the child's questions about school.

Practice needed survival skills while the school has no children in it. Teach the child the visual cues he needs to find the classroom, lunchroom, and washroom (e.g. walk by the music room and the library and your room is next). Visit the washrooms and help the child to feel comfortable with the sounds, smells and behaviors needed to use the washroom. Practice whatever classroom method he will need to use to be able to ask to go to the bathroom.

Early in the school year, take a picture of each of the other children in the class so that the child can learn their names at home. These can also be used to help practice social interactions so that the child can practice "talking" to the picture of a child who he knows, to ask him to play, share a toy, etc. (Parental permission will have to be gained before pictures are used of individual children.)

Watch the procedures used within the school for the activities that occur throughout the day. Develop visual cue cards that will help the child to see the sequence of the activities during the day. Practice at home the skills that are needed within the school setting, such as lining up, circle time, snack time, bathroom time. Develop Social Story™ pictures to help remind the child of the sequence and reasons for the behavior. These stories are useful for them to have at school for the teachers to use if the child becomes reactive.

In early elementary school years, the loud, confusing lunchroom may be overwhelming for the quiet, anxious, withdrawn child. Find the quietest area of the room or an alternate spot for the child. Practice taking clothes and snacks in and out of his backpack. When the child attends all day, discuss what is considered a snack and what is lunch food. Make lunch food that is easy to eat and attain (e.g. unwrap commercially wrapped food and put in a ziplock bag for easy access). Send snacks that the child will eat and that respect oral and gustatory needs. This is important during preschool years since many preschools provide the snack.

To start the school morning in a quiet calm manner, have a predictable morning routine at home. Visual stimulation of TV at home before school may over-stimulate some children so there is a need to limit this entertainment before school. Plan to have the child enter either before or after the school bell, lineups or cubbies routines happen, if noise and personal space are issues.

The activity of "show and tell" presents another challenge in the primary grades. Give the child simple objects to tell about that are precise and small so the child does not have to explain with a lot of detail. Rehearse what the child is going to say before he takes the object to school.

Prepare the child for when holidays from school are going to happen, and prepare him ahead of time for when he will be returning to school. Reminders are needed of the time that bedtime will be, and the daily schedule when it changes to accommodate the return to school routines. Help the child to realize that many of his feelings are the same as other children's. Describe what happened when you first went to school so the child realizes that everyone feels a little anxious about new experiences.

Talking about the school day with the child with Regulation Disorders

Some children with RDSP will not answer direct questions about their day at school or what activities they were doing at school or during play. They appear to see these questions as a threat. Other children have short-term memory problems and cannot remember what they did in the morning or afternoon to tell about it. Questions need to be asked while the child is in the school context so cues are available.

If possible, talk to the teachers about how the day went, and what the child did. This will give information to help initiate conversations so the child does not have to remember or produce all the information. Parents should not expect busy teachers to talk with them every day. Many schools have a daily agenda book that can be used to transfer messages between home and school. By remaining for a few moments in the playground with other parents, the other children may share with their parents and provide clues to the day's activities.

Keep a copy of the school day schedule available and ask about specific events, for example "What story did the teacher read today?" Often asking indirect, general questions rather than direct, specific questions will result in answers, for example "I saw the kids in your class bringing out plasticine animals. That must have been fun. What kind of animals did people make?"

To diffuse some of the personal intensity, use a puppet at home to talk about the day so the conversation is one step removed from the direct experience of the child. Sometimes, sharing personal school experiences to introduce the topics – for example "I remember doing finger-painting. At first I didn't like the feel of it" – will help the child to understand that his experiences are shared by others.

Academic transitions and the child with Regulation Disorders

Within most schools children can expect to move into a new classroom every year. This results in transitions with a new teacher, new routines and at least some new classmates. There are also a number of critical academic transitions that may affect the child with RDSP more than other children.

The change from kindergarten into grade one often signals the increase in need to respond to rules and regulations. There is also an increased need for more sustained attention, printing skills and sitting in a seat, as well as increased focus on the academic tasks of reading, writing and mathematics.

At intermediate grade levels the children are expected to produce more written work and begin to think on a more abstract level. The last years of elementary school bring an increase in social aspects as well as a need for more academic and social independence and further abstract thinking.

Choosing a secondary school is important in terms of the resources that are available to support the child if there are lingering symptoms of RDSP. Although parents will remain the most important advocate, obtaining a case manager at this level will be important to address any remaining learning or social needs and the academic and social accommodations that may be needed.

Teaching approaches for the child with Regulation Disorders

Most children bond with their classroom teacher. The teacher is a surrogate attachment figure for the child. Within the classroom, the teacher can provide the "secure base" that the parents provide for their child at home. However, the child with RDSP may be reactive to the changes and types of teachers that they have. Parents need to have leeway in terms of participating in the choice of the teachers that instruct their child.

Developing a collaborative working relationship with the child's teacher and other school personnel is essential. Parents, teachers, classroom aides and principals need to work together and share ideas of how to adapt to the child's unique sensory and emotional needs. Parents have had years of experience dealing with these issues before the child arrives at school. Problems can be circumvented by arranging to meet with teachers frequently to discuss progress and problem-solving related to the child's needs within the school environment. Adaptability is an important quality (both for parents, teachers and community workers) to maintain when working with the children.

While many children learn by observing behaviors, the child with RDSP often has to have the behavioral or academic information specifically stated. Modeling of the desired behaviors needs to happen in both an explicit (defined and taught) and implicit (role-modeled in contextual situations) manner.

Because many of the children with RDSP have aversive auditory responses, keep instructions brief and simple and given in a soft-spoken manner. Maintain a neutral feeling and voice tone when disciplining the child.

Often the children have problems with attention. Some days they are totally attentive and on other days, or portions of a day, they are totally inattentive. It is often too much emotional effort for them to pull themselves together, so adults have to simplify their environment and calm them to get them through the day. The child can often learn even though he may not be involved in a group activity or appear to be listening. Ignore the child who leaves the group, as long as the child is not disruptive. The child will generally return when he is able. Check with the child individually, after the activity, to see what he has retained. Develop reasons for the child to remain in a circle or story time, for example the child picks out the story, turns the pages or gathers up the sitting pillows. The use of novel approaches to maintain or gain attention in the classroom is important, such as singing the directions to be followed or clapping a rhythm. Some children, however, find singing intolerable and clapping too loud. If the child can tolerate the noise, sound boundaries such as a timer can be used to designate the end of a learning or timeout period. Use a carrel for helping to focus while doing school work or for a timeout so the child can focus on the needed tasks or calm down.

It is important that children with RDSP see themselves as part of the classroom community. Make use of the children's interests and skills to extend their learning beyond perseverative ideas and to help them demonstrate to themselves and others that they have abilities. Offer choices to the child and incorporate his ideas. Use a non-verbal cue picture such as a stop sign or a soldier at attention to point to on the child's desk rather than verbally trying to direct the child back to a task. This avoids frequent calling out of the child's name, which labels the child and his behavior. A culture may develop around the child related to complaints about him that are made by the other children so it is important not to add to this inadvertently by adult behaviors.

If the child has a lower cognitive ability, then adjustments need to be made and instruction given to his cognitive ability. However, do not assume that the children need to start at a lower cognitive level unless they are globally developmentally delayed. Start at an age-appropriate level or use bridging to help them to use their verbal skills to guide poorer motor skills. Children with RDSP often need to see the "whole picture" of what is being described or talked about. While mind maps and other techniques will be helpful as part of a learning strategy, they function better if they know about the whole event or the sequence of steps to complete a task.

Short, specific instructions or questions interspersed with longer, more complex questions often work best.

While most classrooms have consistent routines, seasonal events, visitors, and constructed events add diversity in learning for the child. These changes are often upsetting for the child with RDSP. However, if a teacher or parent is totally consistent all the time, the child may become bored. There is a need for some changes to help stimulate the child to respond in new and different ways and respond to his creativity. The changes have to be made in such a way that it doesn't affect the child's immediate space. If a change is temporary, the children seem more tolerant – it doesn't impact on their secure base. If children are helped to explore the new events from their own perspective (e.g. at Hallowe'en they may be upset by others wearing a mask but not mind putting on a mask themselves) they may gradually learn to tolerate change.

Developing classroom environments for the child with Regulation Disorders

When considering the adaptations needed within a classroom or in classroom routines, teachers need to use a problem-solving strategy. They need to be proactive and, knowing the sensitivities of the child with RDSP that is in their class, consider the possible sensory, motor and behavioral reactions that might occur during any learning event.

By providing a daily "shape of the day" so all children know what will be happening that day, the anxiety that many children with RDSP experience will be decreased. If needed, develop a separate one for the individual child with RDSP if he has a unique schedule. Use visual cues, pictures and reminders for both the sequence of activities and behavior expectations in the class.

Each day, highlight any unusual events and explain what will happen and expected responses. Role-play and practice the response for the child who is anxious or rigid in his need for routine. Problem-solve around how to respond and how to adapt to the new event, for example hands over ears when the fire bell rings, as well as the need to line up. Substitute teachers often increase the distress level for the child – if at all possible, parents need to know ahead of time if the teacher is going to be absent so they can help the child to accept this change before arriving at school.

Placement of the child's seat in the classroom needs consideration. Organize a quiet desk area that any child in the class can use for work away from the class. Children with RDSP often take in more stimuli than other children so need a retreat location to aid concentration. Children with RDSP often do not do well sitting at the front of the class. They do not like direct gaze and often feel over-scrutinized. Place them at the side or back of the class. Allow children to stand at counters or high tables to do coloring, painting, and writing. This will help to accommodate their need for movement during the day.

Adapted equipment may help the child to attend or respond to movement and motor needs. Explore if an inflated Move 'n' Sit seat helps to decrease the need for a child to sit on his legs or move in and out of the desk. If using adapted equipment (e.g. Move 'n' Sit or pencil grips), have more than one so other children can use the equipment too and the child who needs it is not stigmatized. Allow children to use squeeze balls or doodle during listening times to help occupy their hands or to provide deep pressure that is calming to them.

Transitions represent critical events for many children with RDSP. The teacher will need to always be aware of the child's need for warnings, the use of a cue such as an egg-timer to make visual the remaining time, the use of a sequence of pictures to help the child "see" the sequence of activities throughout the day. Be aware of triggers such as lineups and getting belongings that may precipitate aggression. A possible strategy for the child who is reactive to touch or closeness is to be at the front with the teacher holding the child's hand to help guide directional sense and decrease level of responsibility, or to be at the back of or beside the line. This helps eliminate the problem of a child invading others' space or being upset by the space and tactile sensitivity issues that the child has.

Teach all the children in the class about the idea of a personal bubble so they can judge personal space. Utilize small groups or one other person as a partner, not large groups, so the child is not confined by numerous children close to him. Be creative about classroom routines so the child can participate in activities such as circle time. Try two circles – an inner and outer so the child who touches or reacts to touch can sit in an outer area with more space and the child has more opportunity to move. Let the child read from their own book rather than holding and sharing a book with another child.

Events outside the classroom may result in distressed behavior when the child returns to the class. Bathrooms and playgrounds provide two possible situations where the child with RDSP may find aversive stimulation. Allow the child to go to the bathroom without flushing for the urinal/toilet since many children find the flush noise very distressing. Locate quiet spots on the playground and encourage several children to play in this area with the child with RDSP.

If a child is particularly anxious about transition events such as starting school each term, have the child attend only part of each school day, gradually adding time in small increments.

Summary

- Many children enter a formalized school system at the age of three when they first attend preschool or nursery school. This transition from the secure base of a family unit within a familiar environment to the changing staff, children and expectations of an educational setting can be very anxiety producing for the child with RDSP. Parents and educators need to develop proactive strategies that anticipate these reactions at the beginning of each school year and throughout the year as children return after holidays.

- Careful selection of a classroom and teacher that will respond to the individual needs of the child is important. Identifying a receptive teacher and resource staff within the school system who will be available for consultation and support is a critical factor in choosing a school. Information about RDSP and the general presentation of these children, as well as the specific needs of the individual child, classroom modifications and teaching approaches that have been found to be useful, can be provided before the child enters the classroom. Developing a positive collaborative relationship with education staff at all levels will also help ensure that the child receives the most appropriate teaching and resources for his individual needs.

- Parents will need to continue to provide the primary secure base for the child as they help the child to learn problem-solving strategies for new situations, help diffuse anxiety and reinforce positive changes.

Chapter 12

SOCIAL SKILLS AND THE CHILD WITH REGULATION DISORDERS

Integration of sensory and emotional input from the environment may be difficult for many children with Regulation Disorders of Sensory Processing (RDSP). This may affect their social interactions by making them less alert to others' behaviors, facial expressions and verbal interactions.

By age six most children should be able to have a two-way interactive conversation and play in a reciprocal fashion. However, for the child with RDSP the emotional responses and social awareness and conversations needed for group games or team sports are often difficult. A child with RDSP is frequently more socially immature than her peers. Often the child is inflexible and has difficulty sharing toys or play spaces (see Figure 12.1).

Although they want to be within a social circle, they bump and push and alienate themselves. They want to be the leader and if others don't want to follow they prefer to play on their own. Some children are very protective of their own ideas and own secrets. A creative child or a child with high verbal skills may find that other children their age do not understand their ideas or play. They have an intolerance of others' lack of knowledge but they do not have effective skills to communicate to others. "By accident" is a difficult concept for the child to understand and often accidental situations are interpreted as "on purpose" and blown out of proportion.

Parents need to consider their own social skills and anxieties. They may feel anxious about having to always anticipate and respond to areas of concern for their child. The parents may have a social fear of their own related to previous aggressive behaviors of their child. Distress may be created in the parent when the child cannot cope, because of negative reactions of other parents who have implied that they have poor parenting skills.

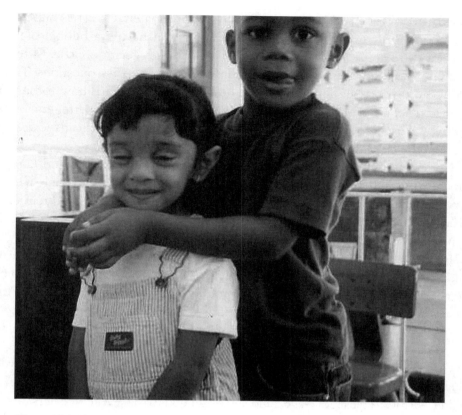

Figure 12.1 Awareness of personal space and boundaries is often difficult for the child with Regulation Disorders

Obtaining support, both professional and personal, that increases and acknowledges parenting skills is important for every parent. Helping the child to develop one good friend versus a number of friends may be the direction to encourage. In the primary years this is easier to do, since by intermediate school years (age ten and beyond) typical children start choosing their own friends and excluding others. The child with RDSP may take a less competent child under her wing. Some children play better with younger or older children than children their own age. Even though they are somewhat uneven relationships, they do help the child to learn and practice social skills and language.

Learning appropriate social skills

Awareness of personal space and boundaries is often a difficult issue for children with RDSP. In their effort to be part of a group or because of sensory needs, they are intrusive or touch others frequently and inappropriately. Use a real bubble (or a hula hoop) to demonstrate and start the talk about having a bubble of space between two people and what happens if one person gets too close. Often the children use a loud bossy voice to share information or to ask questions. Talking loudly can drive other children away. The child needs to learn how to be quiet. Define a quiet time for the whole family. For some children whispering can be very abrasive so use a low quiet voice. Develop a hand signal that means lower your voice, so the child does not need to have verbal reminders.

Understanding the complex verbal and non-verbal behaviors and language that constitutes the social world is difficult for the child with RDSP. There needs to be consistent adult support for the child to "scaffold" or remind and reinterpret social information and behaviors that occur between the more structured classroom and the schoolyard.

It cannot be assumed that the child with RDSP automatically models on other children's behavior or can respond flexibly to the situation at hand. The child may need help to learn at least one script to introduce herself into play situations. Additional teaching is needed to provide responses and behaviors if the answer of a peer is "No" when they ask to join, and how to cope with this (e.g. "OK, well maybe next time").

Additional approaches can reinforce specific teaching of social skills. Develop social narrative stories with two possible endings – similar to the "choose your own ending" stories. The school-age child can be guided to make a choice between two appropriate possibilities. This helps broaden their thinking about making choices. Read library books that demonstrate social interactions and comment on what the children in the stories said to achieve success. Discuss with the child the social behaviors shown in cartoons and children's videos. The use of teaching videos about social skills may help a child to "see" alternative social behaviors. Make videos for social interactions using peers and siblings to act out common social situations.

Family settings provide many opportunities for both specific and incidental learning of social skills and to use strategies to decrease anxiety. Role-model the skill of sharing, and label what is being done. "I am going to share my candies with daddy and you. I am going to say you each may have one."

Because of social anxiety and lack of skills, many children with RDSP become increasingly isolated as they grow up. Develop methods to decrease anxiety such as having a small toy to hold, or encouraging them to look at happy people when in anxiety-producing situations..

By constructing play situations so the outcome will be positive it helps the child to see that involvement with other children can be personally rewarding. Try to find children with a similar ability level and interests with whom the child can play.

Supervise the child while she is playing with other children and intervene before play gets rough or deteriorates. Discuss possible topics of conversation before the visiting child arrives. Initiate play dates even if the child does not get invited back to the homes of others.

For first-time parents, it is particularly important to compare notes with other parents. This helps to develop awareness of the norms in behavior, dress, talk and interests of other children who are the age of the child. Rehearsal of these skills the children need to participate in social activities can then be initiated.

Social Stories™

Social Stories™, developed by Carol Gray, an educator and consultant for students with Autism Spectrum Disorder (ASD), is an approach that uses both visual and verbal methods to help children understand social language and a sequence of social responses.

Social Stories™ are written and photos or pictures drawn to match the pictures and to describe specific topics. The text is used to describe what is happening and why it is happening and to suggest possible solutions for situations that the child may encounter. Each Social Story™ provides a record that the child and adult can refer to for similar events.

The stories help the child to internalize the information by having an illustrated, ready reference and provide a script for self-talk or interactive talk. Initially the child will need to self-talk out loud about how to solve problems in an external fashion, but the goal is to work towards internalized problem-solving. Social Stories™ help the working memory by providing visual and verbal cues. The memory of how to manage responses becomes permanent with use and repetition. Because children with RDSP often see the world as black and white, they need practice in developing a variety of responses. After the child learns one effective response, work on variations so the child has more than one possible response – leading to more advanced problem-solving strategies.

Social Stories™ consist of:

- *description of the topic* (e.g. sharing toys)

- *description of where the situation happens* (e.g. when children come to play at my house)

- *description of the appropriate response* (e.g. children like to play with new toys; it is important to decide which toys I will share)

- *description of what to do if there is a negative outcome* (e.g. if children grab toys or do not share, I will try to ask an adult to help)

- *description of what the positive outcome will be that summarizes and reinforces the information in the story* (e.g. if I share, children may like to come to my house to play with me).

Within the stories use words such as *try to, usually, often* and *may*, for example: "Usually children share their toys", "Often the children will be happy to share", "I will try to ask an adult."

> It may be fun to have children come to play at my house. When the children come they often want to play with my toys. I will try to decide what toys I will share. Usually children try to share the toys with one another. If someone grabs toys or is not sharing, I will try to ask an adult for help. By sharing my toys, other children may want to play with me.

Descriptive sentences are used for much of a Social Story™ with inclusion of other sentence types of perspective, cooperative, directive, affirmative, and/or control sentences (Gray 2005, 2006).

Choosing social activities for children with Regulation Disorders

Inclusion of the child with RDSP into community social events can be successful if preplanning occurs. This will include consideration of the timing, place and type of activity.

Assess the environment before an event – learn the times when many children frequent the playground, what time of day there is more traffic noise, or when is the calmest time for a fast-food restaurant. Have only one other child or no more than three children for a play date, rather than a lot of children, to decrease the noise and increase interaction potential.

Be strategic about the choice of activities with other children that are organized. Organize picnics, potluck barbeques, or activities such as swimming (as long as the child can tolerate noise), where all the children can move about. Have playtimes during the day when the child may be more relaxed and not have stress from the accumulated activities of the day. Activities that do not have many rules (other than safety rules), such as fun on the playground equipment or hiking in a local woods, will increase play success. Choose activities that are interactive but where there are not too many rules and where after a short participation the child can sit back for a while (e.g. card games rather than a long board game). Review expected behaviors, including safety behaviors, before any activity begins.

Select activities that have movement and variety within them (e.g. soccer vs. baseball, clay work vs. painting). If the child is highly motivated to play a sport such as baseball, see if her position can be in an active area such as infield. This will help to keep the child alert and involved. Select activities that are in vogue as well as those that appeal to the child's interests and help the child to have similar experiences as others, as well as have different ones to share and be admired by peers. Supervised activities with another child within the home, such as putting the toppings on a pizza or cutting out cookies, are ways to help children learn to share and interact.

Make sure to have a variety of daily experiences so the child has real content when talking about their experiences. Children will often select computer games to play with a friend. However, these games are quite isolating since usually only one child can play at a time while the other watches. Use computers for interactive activities such as scanning family or friends' pictures to make a collage, not as a choice for peer activities.

Some children are too interactive – incessantly approaching other children, intense in their social responses and with outrageous and attention-seeking behaviors. Frequently it is girls who engage in these behaviors and they may become victims of relational aggression with stigmatization from their peers. It is useful to develop a buddy system by matching a bossy child with a less assertive child. By developing and enhancing the child's physical, social and emotional strengths they can have a legitimate reason to be the center of attention or a leader. The child could be described as having "leadership abilities" rather than being "bossy" if they are given the help to develop the leadership skills in a social way. It is often easy to forget to focus on the positive behaviors and abilities when children most frequently have erratic or negative behavioral responses.

Some children develop one friendship and then are devastated when that friend wants to play with others or moves away. Help the child to interact with several friends so that she has more than one social resource. The parent may need to monitor and invite other children for play dates so there is variety in their child's interactions.

Playgrounds

Playgrounds are highly stimulating and filled with noise and confusion. They are often only partially supervised by adults in a school setting and seldom supervised in community settings. Crowds of children may be confusing or over-stimulating to the child with RDSP. Assess the environment before entering a play space or before setting up a play date with another child.

It is important to locate quiet and calm places for the child within the school grounds or community play areas. Inform supervising adults where these places are and why the child may be standing there.

Develop physical strategies for children to use if they become upset or over-stimulated in the playground area, such as hold onto their thumb, take deep breaths when angry, move away for a quiet time. In the winter, earmuffs can be used to muffle school or playground noise.

Children may have difficulty leaving activities such as the swing during recess play because of their sensory-seeking needs. Limit the access to swings or give lots of warning and stop the play before recess is completed so they can stabilize their behaviors.

Learning of social behaviors needs to be in the moment, at the time of difficulty. At school, if the child has access to a teaching assistant, some of their supervision time needs to be shifted to include lunch and recess to help the child learn appropriate alternative responses during these highly stimulating and interactive times.

Summary

- Understanding the complex verbal and non-verbal behaviors that constitute the social world is often difficult for the child with RDSP.

- Awareness of personal space and boundaries is frequently a challenge for the child and many of her behaviors may be responsive to the child's sensory needs rather than social context.

- Activities that are interactive, action-oriented, and without many rules can be successful with a small group of children.

- Parents will often need to teach the specific social skills required for the event and be prepared to supervise and assist with more intricate social interactions and interpretations.

Chapter 13

MEETING THE NEEDS
OF FAMILY MEMBERS

Meeting the needs of siblings of the child with Regulation Disorders

The following suggestions were given by children age 6 to 13 years old who were siblings of special needs children. The suggestions speak to the needs of the children in the family who may be overshadowed by the more dramatic and insistent needs of a child with "special needs." They are useful reminders that the siblings also have special needs:

- As well as planning to have family time each week, spend special one-to-one time with each child, each day.

- Choose activities in which all family members can participate in their own way – dancing, swimming, drawing, making a pizza, putting pictures in the family album, charade games.

- Ask each child how his day went and to describe something that was fun for the child during the day. Participate in each child's extra-curricular activities.

- Find ways so that every child feels they are the best and not second to the child with special needs. Acknowledge each child's accomplishments. Develop an ongoing "I love you because…" bulletin board for each family member, so the positives become visual (photos, notes, report cards, etc.) and available for all family members to see.

Talking frankly in a non-judgmental way about the needs of the child with Regulation of Disorders Sensory Processing (RDSP) and the time and energy the child takes, is an important discussion for all the family members. Tell the children the "bad stuff" in a way that acknowledges that solutions are the parent's responsibility. Children can tell from worried looks and voices that everything is not "OK" when there is tension related to their sibling. Talk individually to each child and explain, at their level of understanding, about their sibling's needs and disability. Help each child to develop words to say if the child or his siblings get teased because of the special needs child. Search out books that describe how to deal with having a sibling with "special needs."

If the family chooses to attend therapy sessions to solve family interactional or organizational problems, include all the family members during therapy sessions so each family member feels part of the solutions developed.

Advocacy skills for parents of children with Regulation Disorders

To be a competent advocate each parent will need to develop an awareness of the resources for children with RDSP that exist in the local community in the areas of recreation and community programs, health and education.

Recreation and community programs

It is worthwhile to investigate both the programs and supports provided to special needs children for activities offered in community centers. Search out the existence of social skills groups, or groups for gifted children, summer programs, and moms and tots programs that will accommodate a child who may shy away from group contact and may need an adult as a bridging person for a number of sessions. Overnight summer camps are not usually successful until children are well advanced in managing transitions and new routines.

Swim and ski instructors, horse riding instructors, art teachers and music teachers who have experience in working with special needs children are useful resources. Local professional organizations (e.g. the Music Therapy Association) or resources such as the child development center in the community may have names of instructors.

It is important that the child with RDSP try out new social interactions with children and adults when they may know but not be totally familiar with, such as neighbors. Having a neighborhood picnic, lane garage sale or setting up a lemonade stand helps the child to meet and greet new people.

Health resources

Find a doctor, dentist and community health nurse who are willing to learn about RDSP before the first appointment. This will help the visits to these practitioners to be less stressful. Select a dentist and other health professionals who have specialized training in pediatric healthcare. Names of such practitioners may be available from the professional registration board.

Liaison between the physician (pediatrician or child psychiatrist who diagnosed the child) and these other healthcare practitioners is important. These professionals may need the same education about RDSP as the child's teachers or grandparents need. Be prepared to give them written material to read at their leisure.

Education resources

Develop a list of the school board personnel for your geographic area who are knowledgeable about special needs resources. Learn about the process used to request special education resources and understand the legal requirements for provision of equitable education opportunities in the school district. Develop a list of school-based personnel (resource room teacher, school counsellor, principal of the child's school) and the school board personnel (behavioral resource consultant, low-incidence resource personnel, student services within the local school administration). This information is often available on school district websites or through the local school.

Knowing this information will ensure discussion of options with equality of an informed background on both the educators and parents' part. Find out the format used in the school district for an Individual Education Plan/Program (IEP) and prepare a list of the important aspects to be considered for the child that include social and fun needs, and the child's strengths. Take this to the meetings when the school is discussing the IEP for the child – it may help add a humanizing element to the plan.

Attending meetings

Once parents and their child begin to interact with the world outside the home, there will inevitably be meetings to help others to understand the child. By being informed and prepared, parents will be in a position to ask for responses to their questions from others. Take written information about RDSP to leave with the professionals at the meeting.

Before attending a planning meeting, parents need to prepare themselves. However, it is essential to enter the meeting in a spirit of collaboration (not an adversarial approach) if a positive outcome is to emerge.

Sit down and think about what *you* want to get out of the meeting.

Make a list of what you want:

- to get out of the meeting (your goals)

- to ask others at the meeting

- to say to others at the meeting

- to bring to the meeting that supports your ideas or requests – for example, test results, doctor's letters, information about RDSP, strategies that work at home.

Write this plan down and take it and the appropriate materials with you to the meeting. The following strategies can also help you get the most out of a meeting:

- Ask the meeting chairperson to confirm who will be at the meeting, so you know who to expect, their names and positions.

- Plan how you want to be in the meeting; imagine how you want to feel. Think about the one thing you can do to help you feel that way. Take deep breaths and try to relax before you go to the meeting.

- Take someone with you to the meeting. They can be there for moral support or to help remember or write down all the information.

- Write down what you hear at the meeting. This helps you remember what was said, have time to think about it and then return to the topic or ask more questions at a later time.

The language of meetings

Sometimes the language and the official procedures used can make participation in a medical, school or community meeting feel overwhelming. The following suggestions can help you enter a meeting feeling confident and prepared.

To get clarification in a meeting or to obtain a better understanding of what someone is saying
Say: Can you tell me more about that? Can you be more specific?
I don't know what this means, can you please explain it?

If you want more information about a topic
Say: I have a number of questions I would like to ask you – maybe this is a good time…
I'm curious to know how (your child's name) is in (gym time, during circle time).

To give your opinion when you disagree with the information you are hearing
Say: One of the things I've noticed about (child's name) is…(give your opinion/observations).

I see it in a different way…(describe your ideas)
I feel/think it is…

To ensure that actions will result from the discussion
Say: Let me review what we have decided to do and who will be responsible.
I would like a written summary to help me remember individual responsibilities that we have agreed to do today.
Let's plan a follow-up meeting to review our progress towards what we have decided to do.

Ask all your questions – there are no stupid questions. "Keep looking and remembering and talking about the positive changes for your child and family no matter what others say" (advice from a parent of a child with special needs).

Developing parent support systems

Explaining Regulation Disorders

Friends and others involved with the child's family will need education about RDSP, to combat their fear and lack of understanding. Explain the condition as though the child has an allergy – that certain sensory input in their environment affects them in a more extreme fashion than it does for other children. When this happens they have difficulty regulating what is going on within and around themselves and this is often shown by emotional or physical reactions.

Developing support systems

Frequently families do not have their nuclear families around them to help or, even if they are available, the behaviors and needs of the child mean that sometimes even the grandparents feel they cannot cope with the child (see Figure 13.1).

Other parents, relatives or individuals in the community may be negative or judgmental about the parents and their child. The child's behavior often builds a wall around the family and others do not want to visit or invite the family to their homes. The families often have to rely primarily on formal supports in the form of counselors, doctors and emergency help. Develop a support system that includes the family doctor, counselors, and community health nurses. List their telephone number, and all emergency numbers in several accessible areas.

It is unrealistic to expect professionals to provide daily support for families with a child with RDSP. Therefore, it is important to work towards a ratio of three-quarters informal help (family, friends, babysitters), to one-quarter formal help from professionals so that help for everyday problems exists. For such a network to develop and expand parents will need to work on this actively. By being

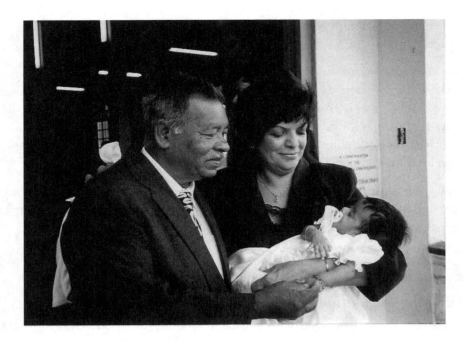

Figure 13.1 Educating grandparents about the child's needs helps them to be a supportive resource

active in the local community, school and block parent organizations, networks of support can be developed.

The staff and organizations within schools can provide another group of support personnel. Enlist the assistance of the school administrator, counselor or teacher to help support the family in discussing with other parents the unusual reactions and reasons for why the child may be reacting that way. Developing a group of special needs parents within the child's school will create a community of support within the school. This could be organized through the Parent Advisory Committee (PAC). There could be representation from this parent group to sit on the PAC to be a voice for the needs of all the special needs children and their parents within the school.

Develop several trustworthy friends who will share babysitting. Select people with like children or who will listen to how the family manage the child and will use similar methods when they care for the child. Help organize a block party, send seasonal cards to neighbors and talk to neighbors when out for a walk, so they know who are members of the family. Have a recent photo and fingerprinting done in case the child gets lost.

For working parents it is important to describe the situation to the supervisor and ask for support in the flexibility for leaving work that may be needed related to the child's "good and bad" days.

A long-term support system can be developed by active participation in policy development, especially within the educational system. Clinicians within the early childhood field are becoming familiar with the diagnosis and treatment of RDSP. Educators are relieved when they acquire information about the difficult path that children with RDSP face, since they too have often been struggling to respond to the needs of the children without any clear direction. Participating with other parents in presentations to district, regional and state/provincial bodies related to the needs of special needs children may result in policy initiatives.

Caregiver survival in the moment

Caregivers take many forms – most importantly the child's parents but also their grandparents, childcare workers, special education assistant, babysitters and daycare workers. We hope these suggestions can provide hope and encouragement to whomever is the caregiver in the moment.

Remember all the positive things about the child and your life with him. Focus on the best things that have happened during the day. Keep a journal of the positive things that have happened each day. Concentrate on optimizing strengths and minimizing weaknesses – your own and your child's.

Sometimes caregivers and educators may feel like giving up, as the task of solving the problems created by a child with RDSP seems onerous and endless. Acknowledge that parents/caregivers/educators may also have sensory overload, feel disorganized and fatigued just like the child with RDSP. To avoid this, be aware of individual and family stress levels, assess how stress is managed within the family or classroom, and develop methods of coping with stress. Recognize "burnout" and take a break. To ensure that problems are solved, define the difficulties on a daily basis to determine patterns of need and then define who can provide help with the problems.

Share both good and bad daily events with a partner/parents/sibling or colleague – whoever will give sympathetic understanding or congratulatory responses. Maintain a sense of humor to contribute to the health of the whole family or working environment. Find something funny to laugh about each day. Remember the siblings – give them extra and special attention since inevitably the child with RDSP will take up extra time.

Looking to the future

It is often difficult to think with a positive perspective about the future of the child with RDSP when each day presents such intense needs and reactions. However, the child will mature, will learn to manage many of his own reactions and all those strengths and abilities will help the child to become a contributing member of society.

So for the present, celebrate the changes in the child and family. Parents often mourn the loss of enjoying a lot of good times with their child. While at times adults can see a really outstanding child, when this positive behavior happens infrequently, the distressing parts seem to be in the forefront. So everyone who is involved with the child needs to concentrate on and recognize the positive attributes of everyone in the family. Families can add these attributes around a picture of each family member and post on an "I love you because…" bulletin board.

Each child needs to have dreams about the future and adults in their lives need to help give the child dreams. Both the child and the adults need to think beyond the distress and the immediate milieu to the possibilities of the future.

Enjoy every moment of relating to this special child – whether at home, in a classroom, in a medical office or on the playground.

Even the most upsetting times become a topic later in the child's life about which to laugh and share memories.

Summary

- Often within a family, or even in a school or community setting, the needs of a child with RDSP become so predominant that the siblings of the child are inadvertently given little attention. Maintaining a balance of time and focus so that all family members feel valued is difficult but worthwhile.

- By developing advocacy skills and support systems at home and in the community, parents can lessen their own stress and can respond with knowledge and a feeling of confidence to the daily challenges that their child presents. Remembering that the future for these special children with Regulation Disorders of Sensory Processing is positive will help everyone to enjoy every moment they spend with them.

Enjoy every moment.

GLOSSARY

Asperger's Disorder: A disorder characterized by deficits in social interaction that are sustained and accompanied by restricted, repetitive behaviors, interests or activities. It differs from Autistic Disorder in that language acquisition is relatively well developed.

Attachment (or attachment security): Signifies a positive, enduring and emotionally charged connection between a caregiver and child. It is part of everyone's life history. A secure attachment typically provides (but does not guarantee) a blueprint for a healthy relational world.

Attention Deficit Hyperactivity Disorder (ADHD): A disorder noted for inattention and/or hyperactivity and impulsive behaviors that must be present prior to the age of seven years. These behaviors are not explained by developmental stages, and interfere with an individual's academic and social functioning.

Autism Spectrum Disorder (ASD): Generally includes several disorders that share some of the characteristics of Autistic Disorder. There is a great variability in presentation with some of the disorders that fall within this spectrum. Examples of the disorder are Autistic Disorder, Asperger's Disorder, and Pervasive Developmental Disorder Not Otherwise Specified (formerly named as atypical autism).

Biobehavioral: A technical description of how biological determinants affect an individual's behavior. This is generally a two-way process where an individual's genes, environment, capacities, and susceptibilities all interact to produce an overt behavior.

Biological rhythmicity: An inseparable internal rhythm that appears to control or initiate various biological processes.

Cry thresholds: Individualized thresholds for cry response that infants develop. High cry thresholds will be noted by a longer time interval before the infant cries (e.g. an infant can look distressed with a crying face but the actual cry will come out after a time interval or an event, such as pain at the injection site). Some infants will instantaneously cry; others will wait for a while or have a shorter first cry sound, and a shorter overall timing of a particular bout of crying. High cry thresholds may be associated with problems in nervous system functioning.

Daily adaptation: Refers to the infant's/child's ability to flexibly respond to daily routines and demands of home life, school life, etc.

Dyspraxia: A specific disorder in the area of motor skill development. Individuals with dyspraxia have difficulty planning and completing intended fine motor tasks. It can affect speech problems, or fine motor activities.

Emotional regulation: A psychological term widely used to denote one's control over emotional expression. Emotional regulation has a central place in self-regulation. It combines the features of emotional modulation, emotional management and expression of emotions in a socially and culturally appropriate manner. It is often used synonymously with the term self-regulation.

Executive functions: Pertain to specific tasks assigned to certain regions of the brain (e.g. prefrontal lobes). These tasks typically involve later evolving, more complex functions of the human brain. They include reasoning, problem-solving, and ability to initiate and stop actions and to anticipate outcomes. Abstract reasoning is also a very important aspect of these executive tasks. The description above is not all encompassing but intended to give a glimpse of complexities involved.

Homeostasis: A balanced state between inter-related physiological, psychological, or social domains that are characteristic of an individual or a group.

Hypersensitive: Reacting excessively to stimuli.

Hyposensitive: Diminished response to stimuli as expected and compared to developmental or group characteristics.

Internal regulation: Suggests that balance is achieved within the inherent capacities or physiological responses (e.g. emotion, behavior, sleep, appetite mechanisms) without input from external resources. For example, internal regulation of emotions for a child suggests the child is trying to control emotions by using internal resources that might include cognitive ability, use of learned experiences, and culturally taught ways of problem-solving.

Joint attention: Taken in a mother–child interactional context, it is the process of sharing an experience of observing an object or an event and then understanding/anticipating what the other has perceived. This is done by young children by following a gaze or pointing gestures. This ability is said to be very crucial for social interactions, language acquisition, and overall cognitive development of the child.

Limbic system: Can also be described as the emotional brain. It consists of highly inter-related nervous fibers and nuclei that form a ring around the brain stem. These structures within the limbic system are responsible for connections with the endocrine system, memory functions, and regulation of the autonomic nervous system that controls heart rate, sexual activity, sleep and blood pressure.

Multisystem Developmental Disorder: A disorder described in a classification system known as DC: 0–3R diagnostic system. This descriptive term is used for infants who have significant impairment in forming social relationships with primary caregivers, as evidenced by their inability in developing meaningful communication (preverbal and verbal). Sometimes they have difficulty in motor planning and processing of sensations (auditory, visual, proprioceptive, vestibular, and tactile).

Neuroadaptive: Adaptation of neural systems to stimuli, or presence of a substance (metabolite). Usually used in connection with conditions such as cocaine addiction, where neural pathways might be speculated as adapting to this ingested substance, or alteration of neural receptors occurring due to a new stimuli (ingested substance), over time.

Neurodevelopmental: Suggests side-by-side and overlapping functions of a child's development that is seen overtly by neurological development, and also suggests how, when this process does not go as smoothly as expected, certain disorders emerge. For example, Attention Deficit Disorder is well known to be a neurodevelopment disorder. There are links between development and intrinsic neurological factors within the brain of the individual child with ADHD.

Neuron: A highly specialized basic unit of the nervous system, a cell that has specific functions.

Parasympathetic pathways: The part of the human nervous system that is concerned with the conservation of the body's energy and resources during relaxed states.

Perception: Awareness of the environment through physical sensation as well as insight or intuitive judgment.

Pruning: A concept applied to paring (removing non-functional neurons).

Psychophysiology: Study of physiological functions (e.g. heart rate, hormonal secretion) associated with psychological (mental, emotional and cognitive) phenomena.

Scaffolding: Provision of a temporary base of information on which further capacities of the child are built, enhanced or supported.

Self-regulation: The essential building block for children's emotionally adaptive behavior and personality characteristics. It is the capacity to regulate one's emotions and behavior to the demands of a particular situation.

Sympathetic dominance: Overriding the parasympathetic system that is usually in opposition to the sympathetic system. As the parasympathetic system has an inhibitory function, with sympathetic dominance this function is underplayed.

Sympathetic system: Along with the parasympathetic system, the sympathetic system constitutes two arms of the autonomic nervous system that is not within our voluntary control. They differ functionally from each other. The sympathetic system produces flight/fight reactions in organs preparing to deal with emergency situations. The parasympathetic system inhibits these reactions. The response of any organ depends upon the stimuli received from each system, and how they react together.

Synapse: The minute space between a nerve cell and another nerve cell that is the seat of action where nerve impulses are passed from one another (with the help of neurotransmitters).

Temperament: Relatively stable characteristics of hard-wired inborn features that determine a child's approach to the external world. It is customary to refer to temperament as hard to please, slow to warm up and easy temperament.

Vagal tone: A physiological process and a marker of stress vulnerability. Indirectly it refers to impulses from the vagus nerve that produces inhibition of the heartbeat.

REFERENCES

American Psychiatric Association (2000) *Diagnostic and Statistical Manual of Mental Disorders (DSM-IV-TR) Fourth Edition (Text Revision)*. Arlington, VA: American Psychiatric Publishing.

Aquilla, P. (2000) *Understanding Sensory Integration*. Workshop presentation, Vancouver, British Columbia.

Ayers, A.J. (1994) *Sensory Integration and the Child*. Los Angeles, CA: Western Psychological Services.

Bagnato, S.J., Neisworth, J.T., Salvia, J.J. and Hunt, F.M. (1999) "The Temperament and Atypical Behaviour Scale (TABS) Manual for the Temperament and Atypical Behaviour Scale." In J.T. Neisworth (ed) *Early Childhood Indicators of Developmental Dysfunction*. Baltimore, MD: Paul H. Brookes Publishing Company.

Becker, K., Holtmann, M., Laucht, M. and Schmidt, M.H. (2004) "Are regulatory problems in infancy precursors of later hyperkinetic symptoms?" *Acta Paediatrica 93*, 1463–1469.

Buss, K.A. and Goldsmith, H.H. (1998) "Fear and anger regulation in infancy: effects on the temporal dynamics of affective expression." *Child Development 69*, 359–374.

Calkins, S.D. (2000) "Physiological and behavioural regulation in two year old children with aggressive/destructive behaviour problems." *Journal of Abnormal Child Psychology 2*, 103–118.

Calkins, S.D. and Howse, R.B. (2004) "Individual Differences in Self-Regulation: Implications for Childhood Adjustment." In P. Philippot and R.S. Feldman (eds) *The Regulation of Emotion*. Mahwah, NJ: Lawrence Erlbaum Associates, Inc. Publishers.

Cesari, A., Maestro, S., Cavallaro, C., Chilosi, A. *et al.* (2003) "Diagnostic boundaries between Regulatory and Multisystem Developmental Delay: a clinical study." *Infant Mental Health Journal 14*, 4, 330–343.

Chess, S. and Thomas, A. (1996) *Temperament Theory and Practice*. New York: Brunner/Mazel.

Cole, P.M., Martin, S.E. and Dennis, T.A. (2004) "Emotion regulation as a scientific construct: methodological challenges and directions for child developmental research." *Child Development 75*, 2, March/April, 317–333.

Cramer, B. (1976) "The parent–child relation as an object of psychotherapy." *Revue de neuropsychiatrie infantile et d'hygiene mentale de l'enfance 24*, 9, 453–460.

DeGangi, G.A. (2000) *Pediatric Disorders of Regulation in Affect and Behaviour*. San Diego, CA: Academic Press.

DeGangi, G.A., Breinbaur, C., Roosevelt J.D., Porges, S. and Greenspan, S. (2000) "Prediction of childhood problems at three years in children experiencing disorders of regulation during infancy." *Infant Mental Health Journal 21*, 3, 156–175.

DeGangi, G.A., Lourie, R.S., Sickel, R.Z., Weiner, A.S. and Kaplan, E.P. (1996) "Fussy babies: To treat or not to treat?" *British Journal of Occupational Therapy 59*, 10, 457–464.

DeGangi, G.A., Poisson, S., Sickel, R.Z. and Weiner, A.S. (1995) *Infant-Toddler Symptom Checklist: Long Version*. Tucson, AZ: Therapy Skill Builders.

DeGangi, G.A., Porges, S.W., Sickel, R.Z. and Greenspan, S.I. (1993) "Four year follow-up sample of regulatory disordered infants." *Infant Mental Health Journal 14*, 4, 330–343.

Dipietro, J.A. (2001) "Fetal Neurobehavioural Assessment." In L.T. Singer and P.S. Zeskind (eds) *Biobehavioural Assessment of the Infant*. New York: Guilford Press.

Dunn, W. (1999) *Sensory Profile*. San Antonia, TX: The Psychological Corporation, Harcourt Assessment Inc.

Dunn, W. (2005) *Dunn's Quadrant Model (Updating our Understanding of Sensory Processing)*. Internet communication www.harcourtassessment.com.

Dunn, W. and Daniels, D. (2002) *Infant/Toddler Sensory Profile*. San Antonia, TX: Therapy Skill Builders, Harcourt Assessment Inc.

Erickson, M.F. (1999) *Infants, Toddlers, and Families: A Framework for Support and Intervention*. New York: Guilford Press.

Feldman, R., Weller, A., Sirota, L. and Eidelman, A.I. (2002) "Skin to skin contact (Kangaroo care) promotes self-regulation in premature infants: sleep-wake cyclicity, arousal modulation, and sustained exploration." *Developmental Psychology 38*, 194–207.

Forsyth, B.W.C. and Canny, P.F. (1991) "Perceptions of vulnerability 3 years after problems of feeding and crying behaviour in early infancy." *Pediatrics 88*, 757–763.

Fox, N.A. (2004) "Temperament and early behaviour form social behaviour." *Annals of New York Academy of Science 1038*, 171–178.

Ghaem, M., Armstrong, K.L., Trocki, O., Cleghorn, G.J. *et al.* (1998) "The sleep patterns of infants and young children with gastro-oesophageal reflux." *Journal of Paediatric Child Health 34*, 160–163.

Gray, C. (2005) *Making Friends and Managing Feelings*. Conference presentation with Attwood, T. Vancouver, British Columbia.

Gray, C. (2006) Personal correspondence.

Greenspan, S.I., DeGangi, G.A. and Weider, S. (2001) *The Functional Emotional Assessment Scale (FEAS) for Infancy and Early Childhood: Clinical and Research Applications*. Bethesda, MD: Interdisciplinary Council on Developmental and Learning Disorders.

Greenspan, S.I. and Weider, S. (1998) *The Child With Special Needs Encouraging Intellectual and Emotional Growth*. Reading, MA: Addison-Wesley.

Hume, R.F., O'Donnell, K.J., Stanger, C.L., Killam, A.P. and Gingras, J.L. (1989) "In utero cocaine exposure: observations of fetal behavioural state may predict neonatal outcome." *American Journal of Obstetrics and Gynecology 161*, 685–690.

Huttenlocher, P.R. (1994) "Synaptogenesis in the human cerebral cortex." In G. Davidson and K.A. Fischer (eds) *Human Behaviour and the Developing Brain*. New York: The Guilford Press.

James-Roberts, I. (1991) "Persistent infant crying." *Archives of Disease in Children 66*, 5, 653–655.

James-Roberts, I. and Halil, T. (1991) "Infant crying patterns in the first year: normal community and clinical findings." *Journal of Child Psychology and Psychiatry 32*, 951–968.

Juffer, F., Bakermans-Kranenburg, M.J. and Van Ijzendoom, M.H. (2005) "The importance of parenting in the development of disorganized attachment: evidence from a preventive intervention study in adoptive families." *Journal of Child Psychology and Psychiatry 46*, 263–274.

Karen, R. (1994) *Becoming Attached: Unfolding the Mystery of the Infant-Mother Bond and Its Impact on Later Life.* New York: Warner Books, Inc.

Kirjavainen, J., Kirjavainen, T., Huhtala, V., Lehtonen, L. *et al.* (2001) "Infants with colic have a normal sleep structure at two and seven months of age." *Journal of Paediatrics 138*, 218–223.

Kutcher, S.P. (1997) *Child and Adolescent Psychopharmacology.* Philadelphia: W.B. Saunders Company.

Laplanche, J. and Pontalis, J.B. (1973) *The Language of Psychoanalysis.* New York: W. W. Norton and Company.

Lester, B.M. and Boukydis, C.F. (1990) "No Language but a Cry." In H. Papousek, J. Jurgens and M. Papousek (eds) *Nonverbal Vocal Communication: Comparative and developmental approaches.* New York: Cambridge University Press.

Lieberman, A.F. and Pawl, J.H. (1993) *Handbook of Infant Mental Health.* New York: Guilford Press.

Lyons-Ruth, K., Alpern, L. and Repacholi, B. (1993) "Disorganized infant attachment classification and maternal psychosocial problems as predictors of hostile-aggressive behaviour in the preschool classroom." *Child Development 64*, 572–585.

Main, M. and Hesse, E. (1990) "Parents' Unresolved Traumatic Experiences are Related to Infant Disorganized Attachment Status: Is Frightened and/or Frightening Parental Behaviour the Linking Mechanism?" In M. Greenberg, D. Cicchetti and E.M. Cummings (eds) *Attachment in Preschool Years: Theory, Research and Intervention.* Chicago, IL: University of Chicago Press.

McDonough, S.C. (1995) "Promoting positive early parent-infant relationships through interaction guidance." *Child and Adolescent Psychiatric Clinics of North America 4*, 3, 661–672.

McKenna, J.J., Thoman, E.B., Anders, T.F., Sadeh, A. *et al.* (1993) "Infant-parent co-sleeping in an evolutionary perspective: Implications for understanding infant sleep development and the sudden infant death syndrome." *Sleep 16*, 263–282.

Ottenbacher, K. (1982) "Sensory integration therapy: affect or effect." *American Journal of Occupational Therapy 36*, 571–578.

Papousek, M. (2000) "Use of video feedback in parent-infant counseling and psychotherapy." *Praxis der Kinderpsychologie und Kinderpsychiatrie 49*, 611–627.

Papousek, M. (2005) "Regulation Disorders in early childhood: Family physician counseling for crying, sleeping and feeding disorders." *Fortschritte der Medizin 147*, 32–38.

Porges, S., Doussard-Roosevelt, J.A., Portales, A.L. and Greenspan, S.I. (1996) "Infant regulation of the vagal 'brake' predicts child behaviour problems: A psychobiological model of social behaviour." *Developmental Psychobiology 29*, 8, 697–712.

Reebye, P. (1996) *The Role of an Infant Psychiatrist in an ADHD Team.* Poster presentation, World Infant Mental Health Conference Tampere, Finland.

Reebye, P., Panikkar, H., Clark, S., Edmison, S. and Stalker, A. (2000) *Autism Spectrum Study: Accuracy of Early Diagnosis and Stability of Diagnosis in a Prospective Analysis.* Unpublished.

Reebye, P. and Stalker, A. (2003) *Five Years Experience with Parenting Groups for Children with Regulation Disorders in British Columbia.* Poster, Early Years Conference, Vancouver, British Columbia.

Richman, N. (1981) "A community survey of one to two year olds with sleep disruption." *Journal of American Academy of Child Psychiatry 20*, 281–291.

Schneider, R. and Robin, A.L. (1973) "The Turtle Technique to Control Impulsive Aggression." In D.M. Gelfand, W.R. Jenson and C.J. Drew (eds) (1982) *Understanding Child Behaviour Disorders.* New York: Holt Rinehart and Winston.

Schore, A. (1994) *Affect Regulation and the Origin of the Self: The Neurobiology of Emotional Development*. Hillsdale, NJ: Lawrence Erlbaum Associates.

Schore, A. (2003) *Affect Regulation and the Repair of the Self*. New York: W.W. Norton and Company.

Siegel, D.J. (1999) *The Developing Mind: Toward a Neurobiology of Interpersonal Experience*. New York: The Guilford Press.

Simonik, D.K., Robinson, S.R. and Smotherman, W.P. (1993) "Cocaine alters behaviour in the rat fetus." *Behavioural Neuroscience 107*, 867–875.

Sroufe, L.A. (1999) Quoted in D.J. Siegel (1999) *The Developing Mind: Toward a Neurobiology of Interpersonal Experience*. New York: The Guilford Press.

Stern, D. (1985) *The Interpersonal World of the Infant: A View from Psychoanalysis and Developmental Psychology*. New York: Basic Books.

Streissguth, A.P. and LaDue, R.A. (1987) "Fetal alcohol: Teratogenic causes of developmental milestones." *Monograph of the American Association of Mental Deficiency 8*, 132.

Tirosh, E., Bendrian, S.B., Golan, G., Tamir, A. and Dar, M.C. (2003) "Regulation disorders in Israeli infants: epidemiologic perspectives." *Journal of Child Neurology 18*, 11, 748–754.

Weider, S. (1997) "Creating connections: intervention guidelines for increasing interaction with children with Multisystem Developmental Disorder (MSDD)." *Zero to Three Journal*, April/May, 19–27.

Weider, S. and Greenspan, S.I. (2003) "Climbing the symbolic ladder in the DIR model through floortime/ interactive play." *Autism 7*, 425–435.

Yack, E., Sutton, S. and Aquilla, P. (2002) *Building Bridges Through Sensory Integration*. Las Vegas, NV: Sensory Resources.

Zeanah, C.H. and Larrieu, J.H. (1998) "Intensive intervention for maltreated infants and toddlers in foster care." *Child and Adolescent Psychiatric Clinics of North America 7*, 2, 357–371.

ZERO TO THREE (1994) *Diagnostic Classification of Mental Health and Developmental Disorders of Infancy and Early Childhood*. Arlington, VA: National Center for Clinical Infant Programs.

ZERO TO THREE (2005) *Diagnostic Classification of Mental Health and Developmental Disorders of Infancy and Early Childhood: Revised Edition (DC: 0–3R)*. Washington, DC: ZERO TO THREE Press.

RESOURCES

Assessment tools

Bagnato, S.J., Neisworth, J.T., Salvia, J.J. and Hunt, F.M. (1999) "The Temperament and Atypical Behaviour Scale (TABS) Manual for the Temperament and Atypical Behaviour Scale." In *Early Childhood Indicators of Developmental Dysfunction*. Baltimore, MD: Paul H. Brookes Publishing Company.

DeGangi, G.A., Poisson, S., Sickel, R.Z. and Weiner, A.S. (1995) *Infant–Toddler Symptom Checklist: Long Version*. Tucson, AZ: Therapy Skill Builders.

Dunn, W. (1999) *Sensory Profile*. San Antonia, TX: Psychological Corporation, Harcourt Assessment Inc.

Dunn, W. and Daniels, D. (2002) *Infant/Toddler Sensory Profile*. San Antonia, TX: Harcourt Assessment Inc.

Greenspan, S.I., DeGangi, G.A. and Weider, S. (2001) *The Functional Emotional Assessment Scale (FEAS) for Infancy and Early Childhood: Clinical and Research Applications*. Bethesda, MD: Interdisciplinary Council on Developmental and Learning Disorders.

Developmental Coordination Disorder

www.fhs.mcmaster.ca/canchild – CanChild Centre for Childhood Disability Research is a multidisciplinary team of researchers working within the McMaster University Health Sciences faculty to develop evidence-based rehabilitation practices. This site provides information for both families and service providers, researchers and students on numerous physical medicine topics.

Developmental levels

Crary, E. (1990) *Pick Up Your Socks and Other Skills Growing Children Need*. Seattle WA: Parenting Press.

Schafer, C.E. and DiGeronimo T.F. (2000) *Ages and Stages: A Parent's Guide to Normal Childhood Development*. New York: Wiley & Sons.

www.zerotothree.org – The ZERO TO THREE website covers infant brain development and general child development during the first three years of life.

Toilet training

Von Konigslow, A.W. (1985) *Toilet Tales*. Buffalo NY: Annick Press. An amusing book to read to children while they are sitting on the toilet.

www.kidsgrowth.com – A site for parents developed by pediatricians that provides parenting resources in the areas of development, medical conditions, milestones, and parenting skills.

Eating, food sensitivities and oral motor needs

DeGangi, G. (2000) *Pediatric Disorders of Regulation in Affect and Behavior*. San Diego, CA: Academic Press.

Satter, E. (1987) *How to Get Your Kid to Eat… But Not Too Much*. Palo Alto, CA: Bull Publishing Company.

Sleep patterns

Lite, L. (1996) *A Boy and a Bear: The Children's Relaxation Book*. Florida: Specialty Press Inc.

Munsch, R. (1996) *Love You Forever*. Willowdale, ON: Firefly Books Ltd. A book with repetition and a soothing story that children enjoy hearing at bedtime.

Sadeh, A. (2001) *Sleeping Like a Baby*. New Haven, CT: Yale University Press.

www.med.umich.edu/1libr/pa/pa_btoilbas_hhg.htm – The University of Michigan Health System child and adolescent health section also provides information about sleep problems and prevention from birth to two years and a resource list of children's goodnight books and books for parents and clinicians about sleep disorders.

Floor Time

Greenspan, S.I. and Weider, S. (1998) *The Child With Special Needs: Encouraging Intellectual and Emotional Growth*. Reading, MA: Addison-Wesley.

www.stanleygreenspan.com – Dr. Greenspan is a practicing child and adolescent psychiatrist and psychoanalyst who has researched and written extensively on the prevention of emotional and developmental disorders in infants and children. He is chair of the Interdisciplinary Council on Developmental and Learning Disorders (ICDL): www.ICDL.com – a useful site that gives information on strategies for working with children with emotional and developmental disorders.

Sensory integration resources

Koomar, J., Kranowitz, C. and Szklut, S. (2005) *Answers to Questions Teachers Ask About Sensory Integration*. Las Vegas, NV: Sensory Resources. Forms, checklists and practical suggestions for helping children in the classroom are included in this book.

Kranowitz, C.S. (1998) *The Out-of-Sync Child: Recognizing and Coping with Sensory Processing Disorder*. New York, NY: The Berkley Publishing Group. Lots of "How to tell if your child has a problem with…" and information on understanding, managing, and helping a child to overcome sensory integration challenges. Videos are also available on information in *The Out-of-Sync Child*.

Kranowitz, C.S. (2003) *The Out-of-Sync Child Has Fun*. New York, NY: The Berkley Publishing Group. Activities and ideas to help provide sensory responsive activities for children.

Yack, E., Sutton, S. and Aquilla, P. (2002) *Building Bridges through Sensory Integration*. Las Vegas, NV: Sensory Resources. Multiple practical suggestions for management of children with Regulation Disorders, autism and PDD-NOS are provided in this book.

www.premier.ca – The Premier catalog carries chewable plastic.

www.schoolspecialty.ca – Sensory Solutions. This catalog has a treasure chest of all things sensory – from specialized gym equipment to fidget toys.

www.sinetwork.org – Information developed and collected by the Sensory Integration Resource Center is shared on this site.

Social Stories™ and language resources

Gray, C. and White, A.L. (2003) *My Social Stories Book*. London: Jessica Kingsley Publishers. A series of Social Stories™ that address behaviors in self-care, home and the community.

www.CriticalThinking.com – Critical Thinking provides a catalog of games and resources to help children expand their reasoning, memory and organization abilities.

www.linguisystems.com – LinguiSystems provides a catalog of language development and social skills resources.

www.socialthinking.com – This website is developed by Michelle Garcia Winner, a speech and language therapist and educator who has developed an approach to help children develop perspective-taking and social skills.

www.thegraycenter.org – The Gray Center for Social Learning and Understanding includes information about Social Stories™ as written by Carol Gray. Staff will read and make suggestions for Social Stories™ developed by parents.

Behavioral management

McCarney S.B. and Bauer, A.M. (1990) *Parent's Guide Solutions to Today's Most Common Behaviour Problems in the Home*. Columbia, MO: Hawthorne Educational Services Inc. This book provides multiple suggestions for common behavioral and attention problems. There are enough strategies to customize adult response to the individual child.

Phelan, T. (2003) *1–2–3 Magic: Effective Discipline for Children 2 to 12*. Chicago, IL: Independent Publisher Group. Also available in video or DVD, this behavioral management approach provides a positive strategy to help parents be consistent and calm when disciplining a child and is effective with most children.

www.freespirit.com – Free Spirit Publishing Company publishes a series of books both in board form and paperback on management of behaviours such as hitting (*Hands are Not for Hitting*, Agassi, M.), and unkind language (*Words are Not for Hurting*, Verdick, E.), bullying and other negative behaviors.

SUBJECT INDEX

AUTHOR INDEX